The Making of Modern Psychiatry

The Making of Modern Psychiatry

Ronald Chase

Cover image: A motor neuron from the ventral horn of the spinal cord (unknown species). Drawn by Otto Deiters in 1865, it is one of the first accurate representations of a nerve cell.

Logos Verlag Berlin

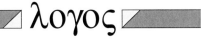

Bibliographic information published by the Deutsche Nationalbibliothek
The Deutsche Nationalbibliothek lists this publication in the Deutsche
Nationalbibliografie; detailed bibliographic data are available
on the Internet at http://dnb.d-nb.de .

ISBN 978-3-8325-4718-9

Logos Verlag Berlin GmbH
Comeniushof, Gubener Str. 47,
10243 Berlin
Germany
Tel.: +49 (0)30 42 85 10 90
Fax: +49 (0)30 42 85 10 92
INTERNET: https://www.logos-verlag.com

For Jack and Niko, with Grandpa's love

Contents

Introduction

Psychiatry is the medical field that deals with mental illness. A woman who finds herself depressed and anxious will seek help from a psychiatrist. A young man who hears voices when no one is present, speaks incoherently on occasion and declines all social invitations may likewise go to a psychiatrist, or be taken to one by his mother. The psychiatrist will interview the person, order some basic medical tests, and perhaps review a brain scan. Once the psychiatrist has diagnosed a specific disorder, treatment begins. Most patients are told to take a drug targeting some specific area of the brain or some specific neural pathway. New drugs are constantly being developed, in many cases by psychiatrist-scientists with expertise in genetics, neuroscience and related biomedical fields. This is modern psychiatry. It developed gradually, beginning in the second half of the nineteenth century.

Everyone is familiar with the great medical discoveries of the nineteenth century – antiseptic surgery, x-rays, vaccines, general anesthetics. Psychiatry had no such discoveries, at least none in the usual sense of the word. Nineteenth century psychiatry saw advances, but few came from the laboratory. Instead, the history of psychiatry in the nineteenth century is mostly the history of ideas and the men (only men) who came up with them. By promoting the idea that insanity is a disease, not a moral punishment or a social deviance, these men lessened stigma and improved patient care. By demonstrating that madness is not unitary, but rather a diverse group of separate illnesses, they instituted major changes in psychiatric diagnosis. And, with the idea of bringing science into psychiatry, they broke ground for the molecular, genetic and neurobiological findings that now offer real hope for better treatments.

Before psychiatry, there was simply medicine, and from its beginning, a small minority of physicians specialized in mental illnesses. In the period from the Renaissance up until the beginning of the nineteenth century, physicians provided services to individuals and families, but there was not yet a medical field of psychiatry. There were no hospitals reserved for psychiatric patients and no professors of psychiatry in universities. Patients, usually described as "mad", were kept at asylums located far from cities.

They received custodial care, but were offered little in the way of treatment. The few doctors whose responsibility it was to manage the asylums pondered the nature of what they confronted. They asked questions. Why do some patients improve with time whereas others fall into irreversible dementias? Can anything be done to help them? Does punishment work? Does reward work? What causes madness? Is the defect in the body or in the mind?

Psychiatry became recognized as a medical specialty when it turned the foregoing questions into scientific questions. This happened first in Europe, and mostly in Germany after the German victory over French forces in the Franco-Prussian War. The new German nation that formed after the war was flush with money and confidence. By investing heavily in transport systems, factories and educational institutions, it fostered a social environment and infrastructure ideal for science and medicine. With scientific projects springing up everywhere, psychiatrists at first observed, then participated.

The central figure in this book is Emil Kraepelin, the man most responsible for creating modern psychiatry. While Sigmund Freud was also highly influential, his contributions were different from Kraepelin's and, overall, less enduring. Whereas Freud adopted a psychological approach to mental illness, Kraepelin became an advocate of biological psychiatry. Freud's patients had relatively mild disorders (neuroses), while Kraepelin's patients had more severe illnesses (psychoses) such as schizophrenia (which he called *dementia praecox*) and bipolar disorder (which he called manic-depressive insanity). Over time, Freud's innovative method of treatment, psychoanalysis, lost favor within the psychiatric profession, even as his broader ideas became absorbed into popular culture. Contrastingly, Kraepelin's classification of mental illnesses remains embedded in the widely used *Diagnostic and Statistical Manual of Mental Disorders*.

Although Kraepelin was the main actor, he was by no means the only person bringing about changes. His support for a science-based psychiatry was shaped by the writings of Wilhelm Griesinger, a German internist who extolled the benefits of basic biological research for medical advancement. As well, Kraepelin's ideas on disease diagnosis drew upon the novel insights of Karl Kahlbaum, a somewhat eccentric and reclusive psychiatrist from eastern Prussia.

Two other men, also associated with Kraepelin, are featured in this book. Bernhard Gudden was Kraepelin's mentor early in his psychiatric career. Gudden was schooled in the old asylum-based psychiatry, but he became a pioneer of the new hospital-based psychiatry. Besides introduc-

ing Kraepelin to clinical psychiatry, he also taught neuroanatomy to Kraepelin's long-time colleague, Franz Nissl. Unfortunately, Gudden suffered
an early, tragic death in circumstances indicative of psychiatry's growing
social power.

Nissl was a psychiatrist who, like many other German psychiatrists at
that time, mixed clinical care with neuroanatomical research. Whereas
Kraepelin relished the intellectual challenges of clinical psychiatry, Nissl
lived to work in the laboratory. He made a few discoveries, but he also
squandered time trying to prove untenable hypotheses. Thus, he was not
nearly as successful, nor as influential, as Kraepelin. Nevertheless, because
of his close personal relationship with Kraepelin, and because he participated in the campaign that demonstrated the brain's astonishing complexity, I highlight his life and work.

Germany was not the only country in which modernization occurred,
nor was neuroanatomy the only pursuit of the scientifically minded nineteenth century psychiatrists. The Parisian Phillipe Pinel and his pupil
Jean-Etienne Esquirol instituted reforms and began to identify and define
specific mental illnesses. The task of diagnosis was to prove especially
troublesome for many psychiatrists, and it became an obsession of Emil
Kraepelin. Also in France, the theory of hereditary degeneration was born.
It was a seductive speculation that seemed to explain the prevalence of
insanity within certain social classes.

Degeneration theory spread rapidly throughout Western Europe, but less
so in America, which was still relatively isolated from European developments. Although Benjamin Rush and Dorothea Dix accomplished important reforms in patient care, Americans did not significantly advance the
science of psychiatry until European ideas arrived in America early in the
twentieth century.

Readers may be surprised to find fulsome descriptions of scientific experiments in this book. I have included them because science is the hallmark
of modernization in psychiatry, and it was not all brain research. Kraepelin, for example, ardently pursued experimental psychology, believing it
to be the key for understanding mental illness. Nonetheless, for most of
Kraepelin's peers, neuroscience was the main attraction.

Before Galileo, it was assumed that all celestial objects circle around
the earth. God's works were perfect and the earth was at the center of
the universe. The telescope changed everything, because it allowed Galileo
to see a different kind of universe. Several centuries later, neuroanatomists
began seeing small nerve cells in the human brain, thanks to newly powerful

microscopes. The outward looking telescopes helped humans find their place in the universe, whereas the inward looking microscopes provided clues to our mental lives.

I tell the stories of the men and their ideas in roughly chronological order, albeit with sidetracks. My account of early modern psychiatry begins in the early 1800s and ends at midnight, New Year's eve, in the year 1899. The final chapter differs from all preceding chapters. It brings nineteenth century European advancements to America and updates them to present day concerns; intermixed with that, I offer my thoughts on the future of psychiatry.

No full-length biography of either Kraepelin or Nissl has yet appeared, although Kraepelin did leave an autobiography of sorts in his *Memoirs*. Elsewhere, the lives of Kraepelin and Nissl are documented in their research articles, letters and administrative papers. Many important works of the nineteenth century were published originally in German, but most have been translated into English; when available, I have relied on these translations.

I am indebted to the intrepid scholars whose research in this treacherous field enabled the present work. Several of their books are listed in the Recommended Readings. The Osler Library of the History of Medicine at McGill University was a great resource for both printed and online sources. I thank Dr. Maike Rotzoll, who hosted my visit to Kraepelin's former clinic at the University of Heidelberg and allowed me to photograph documents held in the clinic's archive. Ursula Voss translated a nearly impenetrable article from the *Heidelberger Tageblatt*, and Rüdiger Krahe helped with other translations. Karen and Gene Brewer reviewed an early version of the manuscript. Special thanks to Volkhard Buchholtz, publisher and editor *außergewöhnlich*. Dorothy Chase was encouraging and supportive from beginning to end.

1 Institutional Reforms

Mental illness may well been present in human communities from the very beginning. Persons portrayed as having bizarre behaviors or nonsensical speech are mentioned in the preserved writings of ancient Greece. Plato thought that such cases arise when passion and appetite gain control over reason. He, together with most of his contemporaries, believed that the gods were behind mental disturbances. Any god can take possession of a person's soul, and if so, troubles will follow. Hippocrates had a different opinion. He blamed poisoning by the accumulation of bile and phlegm, suggesting that "those who are mad from phlegm are quiet, and do not cry out nor make a noise; but those who are mad from bile are vociferous, malignant, and will not be quiet."[1]

Later, in medieval Europe, Church doctrine encouraged a view of madness similar to Plato's. In the revised version, madness was seen as the sign of spiritual possession by devils, witches, sorcerers and werewolves. Affected individuals threatened the community and were dealt with accordingly, that is, harshly.

How communities elsewhere and at other times reacted to having a mentally ill person in their midst, is hardly known. Surely some individuals were physically restrained – in chains for example – to prevent them from harming themselves or others. By contrast, other individuals may have been seen as gifted with rare positive qualities such as fortune telling, healing, or sorcery. These latter persons may have had a relatively high status within their communities.

What to call these persons who behave so differently from the majority? The history of psychiatry is a wondrous thing, as will be demonstrated on many pages of this book. The earliest known term for a mentally ill person was wode, an Old English word that dates from around 1000 AD. According to the Oxford English Dictionary, the word mad (in the sense of a mental disorder) first appeared around 1330. By the year 1384, at the latest, wode had become wood, and it had roughly the same meaning as mad. The equivalence of wood and mad can be seen in a translation

---

[1] Hippocrates, *On the Sacred Disease.*

of the Hebrew bible dated to 1384. There, in the Book of Hosea, chapter 9.7, it is written, "Yrael, wite thou thee a fool, a wood prophete ... for the multitude of thi wickidnesse, and multitude madnesse." From the time of the Renaissance to the end of the Enlightenment (around 1800), mad and madness were the predominant English language terms for what we now call mental illness. One particularly quaint reference to madness is credited to Henry Swinburne who wrote, in 1590, "They did see him hisse like a goose or barke lyke a dogge, or play such other parts as madfolks use to doo." The Oxford English Dictionary lists a remarkable number of synonyms of mad. The exact number, from the fourteenth century to the present, is 168.

After madness, came insanity, which from the start had a legal meaning as well as a clinical meaning. In British courts, an insane person was one whose mental state excused him or her from civil and criminal responsibility. The French equivalent of madness, up until the nineteenth century, was *folie*. In 1801, Phillipe Pinel starting using the word *aliénation*. He thought it more accurately represented the marginal status of mentally ill persons – outcast and largely ignored. After Pinel used the term in the title of his influential textbook, *Traité Médico-Philosophique de la Aliénation Mentale*, it was widely adopted in Europe and America. A German physician, Johann Reil, coined the term, *Psychiaterie*, in 1808, but it would be decades before that word came into general use. The German equivalent of insanity was *Wahnsinn*. The Latin word, *vesania*, had a similar meaning, and it became incorporated in the names of several specific conditions known throughout Europe, for example, *vesanic dementia*.

When mentally deranged (mad) citizens turned unruly or violent in the densely populated cities of medieval Europe, they were confined for security reasons. The Priory of St. Mary of Bethlehem, in London, was perhaps the first institution to serve this purpose. It was established in the thirteenth century as a hospice for all citizens in need, whether they be mentally disturbed, physically sick, or wounded. Records show that, in the year 1403, Bethlehem housed six insane men along with several social misfits. In subsequent centuries, the hospice became increasingly specialized for the custody of insane persons. Its name was shortened to Bethlem, and later still, Bedlam. Taken over by the City of London in 1547, the Bethlem Hospital remained in service until 1948.

Bethlehem was an early example of what later became the common practice of confining mentally ill persons alongside the socially marginalized or physically sick. Unfortunate persons of all types filled the beds in hospitals, almshouses and workhouses. Gradually, toward the end of the eighteenth century, communities in Europe and the United States began reserving buildings and wards exclusively for the insane. These institutions were known as asylums in England and the United States, *Tollhäuser* (fools' houses) or *Irrenanstalten* (mental houses) in Germany, and *hôpitaux* in France. In 1808, when the New York Hospital opened its new building exclusively for psychiatric patients, it was called the Lunatic Asylum, from the French word *lune*, or moon. Psychiatric workers in the nineteenth century were intrigued by periodic or intermittent insanities, and some believed that they were caused by changes in the moon's appearance. The purpose of these early asylums was to confine, restrain, and hide people likely to cause trouble.

At the turn of the nineteenth century, Philippe Pinel, was asked to take charge of a large psychiatric hospital in the Parisian suburb of Le Kremlin-Bicêtre. Born into a humble family, Pinel followed his father and uncle into medicine. As a young man, he participated in the French Revolution. La Bicêtre, the institution to which he was assigned, was already a historic institution, having first opened its doors in the early seventeenth century. In the ensuring years, it served as an orphanage, prison, lunatic asylum, hospice, and finally hospital, which it still is today. When Pinel worked there, it held about four thousand men, mostly criminals and pensioners, but Ward number seven held about two hundred "alienated" patients. Pinel focused his attentions on Ward Seven.

> The halls and the passages ... were much confined, and so arranged as to render the cold winter and the heat of summer equally intolerable and injurious. The chambers were exceedingly small and inconvenient. Baths we had none [of], though I made repeated applications for them; nor had we extensive liberties for walking, gardening or other exercises.[2]

After two years at La Bicêtre, Pinel went to another Parisian hospital, La Salpêtrière, which was even larger. Patients were segregated by sex. Whereas La Bicêtre was exclusively for men, La Salpêtrière was exclusively for women. In 1795, the year of Pinel's appointment as chief physician, it held about seven thousand patients, most of whom were elderly and indigent.

---

[2]Philippe Pinel, *A Treatise on Insanity*, translated by D.D. Davis. London, Cadell and Davies (1801, 1806), p. 53.

Pinel accomplished many things in his long career, yet he is most often recognized as the man who unlocked and removed his patients' chains. True, he did not like chains and true, he removed them when he found them, but he was not the first to do so. That person was Jean-Baptiste Pussin, the manager of the La Bicêtre hospital. Pussin was neither a psychiatrist nor even a doctor. Prior to becoming manager, he had been a patient at La Bicêtre, undergoing treatment for scrofula, an infectious disease of the lymph nodes. Pinel called him "citizen Pussin".

Patients at both La Bicêtre and La Salpêtrière were restrained when disruptive, but otherwise left mostly alone. Some were given the powdered roots of hellebore plants, as earlier recommended by Hippocrates in the fourth century B.C. Hellebore is highly toxic, and even in small doses it causes numerous adverse effects. It was thought to relieve insanity by purging the body of bad substances – usually named as humors – but in reality its only effect on mental illness was temporary distraction. Bleedings were also occasionally performed as an alternative method of purging, until Pinel stopped them. Agitated patients were soaked in baths, either hot or cold. Pinel preferred the so-called "surprise" baths.

Pinel believed that he could cure, or at least lessen, his patients' misery by psychological manipulation. He took advantage of the hospital environment – and the patients' awareness of that environment – to institute a system of rewards, threats and punishments. For example, if a patient kept pulling out her hair, Pinel would warn her that if she persisted, her hands would be locked into gloves. Another patient might be offered better food or a work opportunity if he refrained from shouting. These measures were designed to encourage rational behaviors. Pinel called the approach *traitement moral*.

Unknown to Pinel, a merchant named William Tuke was experimenting with a similar approach in the north of England. Tuke was the manager of a small, local asylum. Like Pinel, he sympathized with his patients' misery and the poor conditions under which they were forced to live. Looking ways to improve their situation, he arranged for accommodations in a large country house. The atmosphere was family-like, and the patients were encouraged to perform simple chores. They were never punished, and good behaviors were rewarded. Tuke's innovations became known as "moral therapy". Despite the similarity between his approach and Pinel's, and the similar names attached to them, they were rooted in different beliefs.

Tuke was a Quaker managing a Quaker asylum. His ideas on the treatment of patients were presumably based on religious, or at least moral, considerations. Pinel, on the other hand, was skeptical of religion. He was a physician motivated by Hippocratic concerns, in particular the search for effective treatments. He was not resolutely opposed to harsh measures; it was simply that he found them less effective than the "moral" methods. The following passage suggests that he took a practical approach, applying physical or psychological measures, as needed, in individual cases.

> ... straight waistcoats, superior force, and seclusion for a limited time, are the only punishments inflicted. When kind treatment, or such preparations for punishment as are calculated to impress the imagination, produce not the intended effect, it frequently happens, that a dexterous stratagem promotes a speedy and unexpected cure.[3]

Also relevant to the comparison of Pinel and Tuke, is the fact that the word moral had mixed meanings at the time, in both French and English. It had an ethical connotation in some contexts, but a psychological or emotional connotation in other contexts. Tuke probably used "moral" in the former manner, to imply kindness, whereas Pinel probably intended a reference to psychological manipulation. Leaving aside their differences, Pinel and Tuke were the two most influential early reformers of institutional care. Their innovations encouraged *both* humane care *and* the possibility of cures.

The influence of Pinel and Tuke extended well beyond their respective national borders. In America, their ideas took root largely through the actions of a single social reformer, Dorothea Dix. While some of her work was directed toward abolishing slavery, curbing alcoholism and broadening voter rights, her greatest devotion was on behalf of the insane, especially those who were poor or otherwise disadvantaged. Her voyage to England in 1836 was instrumental in setting her agenda, for it was there that she encountered Samuel Tuke and his circle of Quaker reformers. After returning to America, she personally investigated conditions for the insane in her home state of Massachusetts. At the time, there were no public asylums or hospitals for the mentally ill in Massachusetts, only facilities privately owned and privately operated. Dix spared no words in her passionately written report prepared for the Massachusetts legislature.

> I come as the advocate of helpless, forgotten, insane, and idiotic men and women; of beings sunk in a condition from which the most unconcerned would start with real horror; of beings

---

[3]P. Pinel (1801, 1806), p. 68.

> wretched in our prisons, and more wretched in our almshouses
> ... I proceed, gentlemen, briefly to call your attention to the
> *present* state of insane persons confined within this Common-
> wealth in *cages, closets, cellars, stalls, pens! Chained, naked,*
> *beaten with rods,* and *lashed* into obedience [italics in original].[4]

Similar investigations and reports followed in several other states, and most resulted in significant reforms. It was through her efforts, for example, that the State of Pennsylvania established its first public "lunatic hospital".

–//–

If Pinel is the father of modern psychiatry, his pupil, Jean-Etienne Esquirol, could be the uncle of modern psychiatry. The two men became acquainted at La Salpêtrière hospital. Pinel was so impressed with the young physician that he appointed him head of the hospital's psychiatric division. After-wards, Esquirol directed a large asylum in the Parisian suburb of Charen-ton. While Pinel was a broadly qualified physician with a special interest in psychiatry, Esquirol, by contrast, was a doctor almost exclusively dedicated to psychiatry. Moreover, he took upon himself the task of modernizing the delivery of psychiatric care, not only in the asylums where he worked, but throughout France.

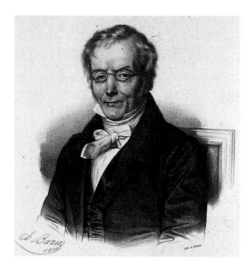

Figure 1: Jean-Etienne Esquirol.

---

[4]Dorothea L. Dix, *Memorial to the Legislature of Massachusetts* (1843). Quotes on p. 2.

Esquirol traveled around France at his own expense, assessing conditions at mental asylums. He was shocked by what he saw. Clearly, the reforms undertaken by Pussin and Pinel in Paris had not gone beyond the capitol city.

> I have seen these unfortunate insane, naked, covered with rags, having nothing but straw to protect themselves from the cold humidity of the pavement on which they are laid. I saw them roughly fed, deprived of air to breathe, water to quench their thirst, and things necessary for life; I have seen them delivered to genuine jailers, abandoned to their brutal surveillance; I saw them in narrow caves, filthy, stinking, without air, without light, chained like wild beasts ... In Toulouse, in a room of about twenty beds, under the roofs, a chain was suspended from the walls bearing an iron belt; the insane, as they ascend into their beds, shake off those chains that will weigh upon them during the night.[5]

After completing three such trips, Esquirol submitted a report to the Minister of the Interior recommending certain reforms. Most emphatically, he wanted psychiatric patients to be cared for at institutions that were designed and maintained especially for that purpose. He wrote that the large dormitories at asylums should be replaced by smaller buildings where the patients could live more comfortably and with improved hygiene. Moreover, he believed that patients should be kept busy and socially involved. He recommended fresh air, calisthenics and physical work.

As part of his travels, he visited the town of Gheel in Belgium. In this centuries-old agricultural community, chronically ill persons – both male and female – lived side-by-side with resident villagers. Esquirol was so impressed with what he saw that he urged the French Ministry to experiment with similar arrangements. In later years, he helped set up a smaller version of the Gheel community at a farm situated close to the hospital at Bicêtre. Also at Bicêtre, he occasionally invited patients to his family home for an evening meal.

Therapeutic farms, of the type established at Gheel, came to the attention of American psychiatrists many years later. When a proposal was floated to build similar farms in the United States, some doctors objected,

---

[5]The quote is from Esquirol's *Mémoire*, presented to the Minister of the Interior, September, 1818 and excerpted in *Mémoires de l'Académie des sciences, inscriptions et belles-lettres de Toulouse*, tome VII (1885), p. 80.

citing concerns over male patients and female patients living in close proximity. Esquirol had written that there were no moral transgressions on the farms and that pregnancies among female patients were "exceedingly rare", but his testimony failed to reassure his American critics. A comprise was proposed, according to which the actual farms would be worked by men, while "a separate establishment, on a smaller scale, [would be] adapted to the females." The female establishment, they said, would be like an "elegant pleasure-grounds" or "merely a large garden."[6] The first American therapeutic community was established in 1913, at the Gould Farm in the Berkshire hills of Massachusetts.

Esquirol advised the Minister that physicians ought to be specifically trained in the care and treatment of psychiatric patients. Moreover, he insisted, the state should give doctors absolute authority and full responsibility for managing affairs at mental institutions. Esquirol argued that while *aliénation* was a social problem, it was also, and principally, an illness. It followed that,

> The physician must be, in some manner, the vital principle of a lunatic hospital. It is he who should set everything in motion ... The action of the administration, which governs the material aspect of the establishment and supervises all the employees, ought to be hidden. Never should the administration appeal a decision made by the physician, never should it interpose itself between the physician and the lunatics or between the physician and the non-medical staff. The physician should be invested with an authority from which no one is exempt.[7]

Responding to Esquirol's reports and recommendations, the French parliament passed a law on June 30, 1838 that called for the building of new institutions – real hospitals – throughout the country. It stipulated that these hospitals should be specifically designed for the needs of psychiatric patients. Requirements with respect to accommodations, hygiene and humane care were detailed. And, importantly, the law clearly stated that *aliénation* was a medical condition requiring medical care and medical treatment. With its many additional provisions, the law was essentially a bill of rights for alienated individuals and, as such, a major achievement for Jean-Etienne Esquirol.

---

[6] John M. Galt, "The farm of St Anne," *American Journal of Insanity* 11:353-357 (1855). Quotes on p. 357.
[7] Quoted in J.E. Goldstein (1987), p. 132.

2 Cutting Nature at its Joints

Pinel's reputation as a reformer obscures his important role in advancing a rational understanding of psychiatric illness. Following the advice of Hippocrates, and in keeping with his empathetic character, Pinel listened carefully to what his patients told him. Like other physicians before and after, Pinel found their symptoms baffling. Recalling his experiences at La Bicêtre, he wrote,

> On my entrance upon the duties of that hospital, everything presented to me the appearance of chaos and confusion. Some of my unfortunate patients labored under the horrors of a most gloomy and desponding melancholy. Others were furious, and subject to the influence of a perpetual delirium. Some appeared to possess a correct judgment upon most subjects, but were occasionally agitated by violent sallies of maniacal fury; while those of another class were sunk into a state of stupid idiotism and imbecility. Symptoms so different, and all comprehended under the general title of insanity, required, on my part, much study and discrimination.[8]

He was intrigued. As a doctor, he knew bodily illnesses. Each was characteristically seated in a particular organ, each had its recognizable symptoms, and many had known causes. He wanted to know if that was equally true of mental illnesses. In attempting to answer that question, Pinel arrived at one of the earliest classifications of mental illnesses. It may seem obvious to us today that bipolar disorder is related to depression but different from obsessive-compulsive disorder, but in Pinel's time such distinctions were not apparent.

Early in the nineteenth century, when Pinel was trying to figure out how to diagnose mental illnesses, there were no departments of psychiatry at the medical schools. Nor was there any academic psychology. Consideration of most things mental fell within in the domain of philosophy. It was generally assumed that the mind is not unitary, but rather a composite

---

[8]P. Pinel (1801, 1806), pp. 1-2.

of several semi-independent functions. This was an old idea. Aristotle, for example, mentions five "psychic powers", namely those responsible for nutrition, appetite, sensation, locomotion and thought. The great German philosopher, Emanuel Kant, recognized three "faculties" of mind: sensibility, understanding and reason. Given this concept of mind as a divided entity, psychiatrists naturally tended to parcel mental symptoms along similar lines and assign illnesses to one or another of the mental faculties.

Plato also weighed in on divisions within the mind. In one of his books, Plato writes of his friend Socrates in conversation with Phaedrus, an Athenian aristocrat. Socrates apparently told Plato,

> We [Socrates and Phaedrus] made four divisions of divine madness, ascribing them to four gods, saying that prophecy was inspired by Apollo, the mystic madness by Dionysus, the poetic by the Muses, and the madness of love, inspired by Aphrodite and Eros ...

Socrates goes on to explain two principles of rhetoric. The first of which is "perceiving and bringing together in one idea the scattered particulars." The second principle is,

> that of dividing things again by classes, where the natural joints are, and not trying to break any part, after the manner of a bad carver. As our two discourses just now assumed one common principle, unreason, and then, just as the body, which is one, is naturally divisible into two, right and left, with parts called by the same names, so our two discourses conceived of madness as naturally one principle within us, and one discourse, cutting off the left-hand part, continued to divide this until it found among its parts a sort of left-handed love, which it very justly reviled, but the other discourse, leading us to the right-hand part of madness ...[9]

So, while madness may appear unitary to the casual observer, the discerning philosopher, by cutting cleanly at its joints, will recognize four types. Whether the actual number is four or something else, philosophers, physicians and regular folks have been looking for the "natural joints" of mental illness for centuries.[10] The result is a complex history of symptoms

---

[9]Plato, *Phaedrus*, sections 265B, 265d-266a.

[10]The branch of medical science that specializes in the classification of diseases is called "nosology".

and concepts that is full of changing definitions, confusing terminologies and national differences of opinion. Only a few scholars have dared enter the tangled mess. The eminent British scholar, German Berrios, plunged in and came up with a book of 565 pages. His *History of Mental Symptoms* is a rich meal, not easily digested.[11] Its tales of discarded terms and seemingly ridiculous classifications serve as reminders of how far we have come in understanding mental illness.

Psychiatric classifiers generally assume that they are working with "real" illnesses, in the same sense as zoologists see zebras and giraffes as "real" animals. Mental illness are not simply abstract notions, the products of scholarly debate. Although there are reasons for questioning this assumption – as will be seen in the closing chapter of this book – few nineteenth century psychiatrists thought otherwise. Instead, they started by identifying and naming the disorders. From there, they proceeded to group the disorders by their apparent affinities, just as zoologists place zebras and giraffes near other mammals but distant from spiders and butterflies. Because psychiatrists believed that the entries in their classifications were real, they took the classifications to be objective accounts of natural order, but that is not likely the case. Psychiatric classifications, like all classifications, are the products of observation, judgment and critical thinking. As such, they inevitably reflect the biases of the classifier.

The earliest classifications of mental illness contained just a few high-level categories and a similar small number of sub-entries. Over the years, the number of entries grew. The current edition of the *Diagnostic and Statistical Manual of Mental Disorders* (DSM-5), considered the standard reference in clinical psychiatry, has about three hundred disorders organized and described in twenty chapters.

The first hurdle faced by a prospective psychiatric classifier is choosing the criteria by which disorders will be defined. There are, first of all, symptoms, which are the subjective experiences reported by the patient. Obviously, such reports will be interpreted differently by different observers. There are also signs, which are the outward indications of disease; they can be seen or heard by any observer and therefore do not depend on the patient's report. Behaviors, speech patterns and physical abnormalities all fall into the category of signs. They tend to be less ambiguous than symptoms and hence more reliable for identifying illnesses. Nevertheless, even signs may not be what their observers think them to be. Phrenology,

---

[11] German E. Berrios, *The History of Mental Symptoms*. Cambridge, Cambridge University Press (1996).

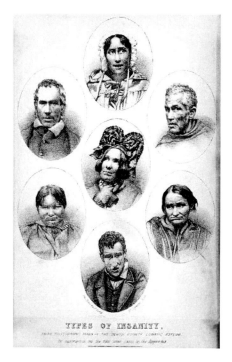

Figure 2: "Types of Insanity, from photographs taken in the Devon County
Lunatic Asylum." [John Charles Bucknill and Daniel Hack Tuke,
A Manual of Psychological Medicine, 1858]

the pseudo-scientific method for assessing a person's mental qualities from
measurements of his or her skull, offers a good example.

The phrenologists relied on an imaginative inventory of mental functions,
or mental faculties. They thought that each mental function was served by
a different part of the brain (albeit limited to the cerebral cortex), and they
invented a map of the anatomical locations. Crucially, they further believed
that as the power of a function grew in any given person, that part of the
brain which was responsible for the function grew too, and pressure from
the swelling would deform the overlying skull. Therefore, deformations of
the skull reflected the vitality of the corresponding brain function below.

Given this set of convictions, the phrenologists palpitated the heads of
clients searching for telltale bumps and crevices. They claimed that they
could discern the strengths and weaknesses of more than forty mental mod-
ules, among which religiosity, love of persons, love of property, mechanical
ability and combativeness. It became a thriving business. And, since ex-

treme measurements were considered pathological, psychiatrists jumped on board offering phrenological analyses to patients and their families.

Physiognomy was a physical method similar to phrenology that was likewise used as a diagnostic tool. Rather than looking to the skull for information about an individual's character, as the phrenologists did, physiognomic practitioners looked at the entire body, especially the face. Already in ancient Greece, learned authors – including Aristotle – wrote that a person's character could be read from an examination of his or her facial features. The idea was revived in the late eighteenth century by a Swiss theologian named Kasper Lavater, who wrote persuasive essays extolling it. Then, an Englishman, Charles Bell, went further. Starting from the premise that the creator had given humans certain sensibilities unknown to animals, and asserting that such feelings are evident in expressions not seen in "lower" species, he concluded that madness is revealed when an individual's expressions are exclusively of the animal type. As he explained it,

> If ... I were to set down what ought to be represented as the prevailing character and physiognomy of a madman, I should say, that his body should be strong and muscular, rigid and free from fat; his skin bound, his features sharp; his eye sunk; his colour a dark brownish yellow, tinctured with sallowness, without one spot of enlivening carnation ... You see him lying in his cell regardless of every thing, with a death-like gloom, I mean a heaviness of the features without knitting of the brows or action of the muscles.[12]

The final step in physiognomic analysis was taken by those who claimed that each type of madness has its own characteristic face. Physicians who added physiognomy to phrenology in their diagnostic tool kits, were thus able to grow their clientele and enhance their incomes.

$$-//-$$

Neither phrenology nor physiognomy held sway with Philippe Pinel. Rather, his approach to psychiatric diagnosis and classification relied almost exclusively on symptoms. There are always symptoms in every disease, but no psychiatrist before Pinel had paid so much detailed attention to them, nor so earnestly endeavored to sort out meaningful constellations.

---

[12]Charles Bell, *Essays on the Anatomy of Expression in Painting.* London (1806), pp. 153-154.

Pinel's classification was the first in a long line of contentious classifications based on symptoms. As explained by the historian Jan Goldstein,

> The classification of data under clear and distinct rubrics was the *sine qua non* of enlightened scientific method in France at the end of the eighteenth century. With respect to psychiatry, that meant – and continued to mean throughout the nineteenth century – drawing up and periodically overhauling ... classificatory systems of mental disease, in which each disease was defined by the cluster of symptoms it regularly presented, and the ensemble was presumed to exhaust all the pathological possibilities.[13]

Pinel occasionally mentioned the cause or causes of an illness, but these speculations neither defined the illness nor influenced the classification. Later authors would place more emphasis on causes, and they added other criteria such as the disorder's course over time and its ultimate outcome. These additions yielded more sharply defined clinical entities, as we will see.

Before Pinel, it was customary to name mental diseases after the circumstances of their onset or the contents of their irrational beliefs. Thus, his predecessors had coined such illnesses as masturbatory insanity, religious insanity and wedding night psychosis. Pinel discarded all those illnesses. Guided by the concept of mental faculties described above, he chose names that captured the fundamental types of psychological disturbance – as he saw them.

Pinel's classification appeared in his textbook, first published in 1801. He began with mania, an ancient term that had a meaning roughly equivalent to insanity. He sharpened the definition by introducing a distinction between two types. The first type, *manie avec délire* (mania with delirium) affected only intelligence, whereas *manie sans délire* (mania without delirium) affected the emotions and basic human drives like sex and hunger, but not intelligence. Intelligence had a different meaning for psychiatrists in the nineteenth century than it does in common speech today. It referred less to smartness than to rationality.

Delirium, like mania, was a word commonly associated with insanity, and this was true in England as well as in France. It referred to states of excited

---

[13] Jan Ellen Goldstein, *Console and Classify: The French Psychiatric Profession in the Nineteenth Century*. Cambridge, England, Cambridge University Press (1987), p. 5.

confusion, particularly when accompanied by disorientation, clouded consciousness and delusion. Then, as now, a delusion is a firmly maintained false belief. Anyone who has had the good fortune (or otherwise) of listening to a patient speak of his or her delusions will likely have thought them highly bizarre. They occur in delirium as well in most other types of severe mental illness. Those delusions that are interpreted by the patient as threatening, are known as a paranoid delusions, and the range of subject matter contained in paranoid delusions is extraordinary. "The patients," one nineteenth century author reported, "believe that they are persecuted, surrounded by spies, tormented by secret enemies who employ electricity against them, tormented by freemasons, possessed of a devil, eternally damned, robbed of their most valued treasures, etc."[14]

That someone could be crazy without losing his or her rationality (mania without delirium) was not an entirely new notion, but some of Pinel's contemporaries were nonetheless skeptical. To convince them that mania without delirium was credible, Pinel described the case of a man detained at La Bicêtre during the French Revolution. When his comrades broke into the hospital to free the political prisoners, Jean-Baptiste Pussin, the manager at La Bicêtre, told the brigands that this particular man, whether political or not, was insane and that he should not be released. The brigands did not believe Pussin, because the man in question made perfect sense when speaking. They liberated him from his chains and shouted "Vive la République!" Upon hearing these words, the man fell into a terrible rage. He grabbed one of the men's sabers and assaulted his liberators. For Pinel, it was a clear case of mania without delirium.

Mania's partner in the traditional language of madness was melancholia. It too has undergone numerous changes of meaning and implication. It initially referred to irrational or lethargic behaviors, but not necessarily sadness as we think of it today. For some physicians, it was akin to dementia. The term took on a more definite meaning in Richard Burton's book, *The Anatomy of Melancholy*, published in 1621. Burton was a cleric in Oxford. He was neither a psychiatrist (there were none then) nor a doctor, but he wrote about melancholy with the insights of a victim. He described melancholic individuals as "not always sad and fearful, but usually so." These persons are, he said, "[for the] most part sad: pleasant thoughts depart soon, sorrow sticks by them still continually, gnawing as the vulture

---

[14]Wilhelm Griesinger, *Mental Pathology and Therapeutics*, 2nd edition, translated by C. Lockhart Robertson and J. Rutherford. London, New Sydenham Society (1861, 1867), p. 328.

did Tityus' bowels, and they cannot avoid it." (Tityus was a vile criminal in Greek mythology. He was punished for attempting to rape Leto, mother of Apollo and Artemis.) After Burton, the popular understanding of melancholia came to be associated with subjective feelings of sadness, but psychiatrists often had their own views.

Pinel recognized melancholia as a type of mental illness, but he struggled to define it. He saw it as a kind of delirium – with delusions – but also as a mood disorder in which the mood might be either up or down.

> Delirium exclusively upon one subject; no propensity to acts of violence, independent of such as may be impressed by a predominant and chimerical idea; free exercise in other respects of all the faculties of the understanding; in some cases, equanimity of disposition, or a state of unruffled satisfaction; in others, habitual depression and anxiety, and frequently a moroseness of character amounting even to the most decided misanthropy, and sometimes to an invincible disgust with life.[15]

Next on Pinel's list came dementia, a Latin word translating as "without mind". Originally, it was yet another term roughly synonymous madness. Later, it acquired a more narrow meaning, referring to a state of mental incompetence and associated with the elderly. A classic description of dementia was provided by Richard Burton,

> [T]hey dote at last ... and are not able to manage their estates through common infirmities incident in their age; full of ache, sorrow and grief, children again, dizzards [blockheads], they carl [act roguishly] many times as they sit, and talk to themselves, they are angry, waspish, displeased with everything, suspicious of all, wayward, covetous, hard, self-willed, superstitious, self-conceited, braggers and admirers of themselves.[16]

Pinel characterized dementia as "the abolition of the thinking faculty". As usual, he wrote at length about representative cases,

> ... a man who had been educated in the prejudices of the ancient noblesse... His passionate effervescence and puerile mobility were excessive. He constantly bustled about the house, talking incessantly, shouting and throwing himself into great passions

---

[15]P. Pinel (1801, 1806), p. 149.
[16]Robert Burton, *The Anatomy of Melancholy* (1621).

for the most trifling causes. He teased his domestics by the most frivolous orders, and his neighbors by his fooleries and extravagances, of which he retained not the least recollection for a single moment. He talked with the greatest volatility of the court, of his periwig [powdered and gathered at the back), of his horses, of his gardens, without waiting for an answer or giving time to follow his incoherent jargon.[17]

The last of Pinel's mental illnesses was idiotism, about which Pinel wrote,

A defective perception and recognizance of objects, a partial or total abolition of the intellectual and active faculties. This disorder may originate in a variety of causes: such as excessive and enervating pleasures, the abuse of spirituous liquors, violent blows on the head, deeply impressed terror, profound sorrow, intense study, tumors within the cavity of the cranium, apoplexy, excessive use of the lancet in the treatment of active mania.[18]

The above description of idiocy is unusual because the simple, one-sentence definition is followed by a long list of possible causes. Pinel was rarely so specific in regard to causes. Here, perhaps, he wished to emphasize the nature of idiocy as an illness of youth or middle age, as opposed to dementia, an illness of old age.

In summary, Pinel's classification of 1801 amounted to this,

- Mania
    - With delirium
    - Without delirium

- Melancholia
    - With elevated moods
    - With depressed or anxious moods

- Dementia

- Idiocy

---

[17]P. Pinel (1801, 1806), pp. 160-161.
[18]P. Pinel (1801, 1806), p. 165.

Esquirol's classification built upon Pinel's, but was more complex and included a few significant modifications. Altogether, he had five varieties of insanity. He included traditional mania (Pinel's *mania avec délire*), but he rejected Pinel's *mania sans délire* because, in his experience every manic patient had some degree of impaired reasoning. Somewhat confusingly, Esquirol introduced two new illnesses, both of which incorporated the word mania in the sense of madness, and yet were distinct from traditional mania and from each other.

The first of his innovations was lypemania, which was similar to Pinel's melancholia, but always "of a sorrowful and depressive passion." His description of lypemania closely matches the present illness of depression. The second new disorder was monomania, a disorder "in which the delirium is limited to one or a small number of objects, with excitement, and predominance of a gay, and expansive passion." Monomania, Esquirol maintained, was a "partial insanity", not just because of the small number of delusional "objects", but also because each patient was insane only in respect to a single mental faculty, of the sort already identified by philosophers. Thus, there were three forms of monomania: affective (emotional), intellectual and instinctive.

In addition to those three *forms* of monomania, Esquirol also mentions several *types* of monomania. The names of the types reflect the contents of the delusions. Thus, reasoning monomania, drunkenness monomania, incendiary monomania and erotic monomania. The last mentioned type must have been especially common, because Esquirol detailed many cases. He, like Pinel, was a keen observer who filled his writings with colorful case descriptions. Because they are so absorbing, one suspects that Esquirol knew that they would be sensational and he encouraged the effect. Nevertheless, few readers would deny the persuasive effect of symptomatic detail in differentiating between various mental conditions. The following description of erotic monomania is a case in point,

> M, thirty-six year of age, is of a nervous temperament, a melancholy disposition, and a small stature. His hair is black, and his physiognomy but slightly agreeable ... He goes to the theatre, and conceives a passion for one of the most beautiful actresses of Feydeau, and believes that his sentiment is reciprocated. From this period, he makes every possible attempt to reach the object of his passion ... The actors, and the husband of the actress, revile this wretched man; repulse, abuse, and maltreat him... He is, at length, arrested in the Tuileries, for having raised his cane,

the dress of this lady ... On every other subject, he reasoned very correctly, his interests were regarded, and his conversation was coherent.[19]

Esquirol's monomania resembles the present-day disorder of obsession-compulsion, especially in its "instinctual" form. He wrote of instinctual monomania that "a lesion of the will exists. The patient is drawn away from his accustomed course, to the commission of acts, to which neither reason nor sentiment determine, which conscience rebukes, and which the will has no longer the power to restrain."[20]

After the customary addition of dementia and idiocy, Esquirol arrived at the following classification of mental disorders,

- Mania

- Lypemania

- Monomania

  - Affective

  - Intellectual

  - Instinctive

- Dementia

- Idiocy

We should linger a while longer on Esquirol's monomania, for it illustrates how messy the cutting up of mental illness can be, especially when it comes to naming the results.

People had been familiar with obsessions for ages, but the concept of obsession as a disease dates only from the nineteenth century. French alienists had several names for it prior to monomania, among which *manie sans délire* (Pinel), *maladie du doute, folie du doute avec délire de toucher, folie lucide, délire émotif and onomatomania*. Notwithstanding Esquirol's fulsome description of monomania, disagreements about the nature of obsession-like disorders persisted for many years. And so did confusion over the names.

---

[19]Etienne Esquirol, *Mental Maladies*, translated by E.K. Hunt. Philadelphia, Lea and Blanchard (1838, 1845), pp. 337-338.
[20]E Esquirol (1838, 1845). Brief definitions of lypemania and monomania, as well as the remaining three types of insanity, appear on page 29.

The story of how afflictions of the monomania type got the current name, obsessive-compulsion disorder, merits telling, because it exemplifies the tortured path traced by so many psychiatric terms. The story begins with Richard Krafft-Ebing, a German expert on forensic psychiatry working in Graz, Austria. He coined the term *Zwangvorstellung* in 1867, and its troubles began soon afterwards. According to German Berrios, an authority on German terminology, the name *Zwangvorstellung*,

> reflected [Krafft-Ebing's] views on the *origin* of the disorder: *Zwang* derives from the high German *dwang* via *twanc* which is the middle high German for 'to compel, to oppress'. The word *Vorstellung,* in turn, meant at the time 'presentation or representation' and had been introduced by Wolff a century earlier to refer to the Cartesian 'idea' [italics in original].[21]

Fine, but later German psychiatrists subdivided Kraft-Ebing's *Vorstellung* into pure mental experiences (obsessive ideas) and precursors of action (compulsions). Then, when *Zwangvorstellung* was translated into English, it came out as obsession in Great Britain, but as compulsion in America. Hence, the now familiar obsessive-compulsive disorder arose as a comprise between the two English translations.

The written works of Pinel, Tuke and Esquirol were known to American doctors and widely respected. So much so, one might say, that the Americans hardly bothered to improve upon them. Only Benjamin Rush, the so-called "Father of American Psychiatry", wrote at length about mental illness and, for the most part, his ideas either mimicked those of his European contemporaries or offered poorly thought out alternatives. It would not be until a century later, after the importation of German advances, that American psychiatry began to modernize.

Rush was an extraordinary person, brilliant of mind, deeply immersed in civic life and prolific. Born in 1745, he served as a top physician in America's revolutionary army, and he signed the Declaration of Independence along with George Washington. Later, as professor at the University of Pennsylvania, he wrote the first American textbook on chemistry, the first American textbook on psychiatry (1812), and numerous tracts on social reforms. Like his European contemporaries, Rush was not actually a psychiatrist, but a broadly trained doctor with a particular interest in insanity, or madness. His unusual conclusions regarding the cause of mental illness

---

[21]G.E. Berrios (1996), p. 141.

and the treatments appropriate to it, will be examined in the next chapter. Here, we examine his classification, which he presented in his textbook.[22]

Rush's classification re-arranges the categories named by Pinel and Esquirol, while adding other disorders and introducing numerous neologisms. He describes madness as intellectual derangement, which he claims comes in two forms, partial and general. Some types of partial intellectual derangement resemble monomania. When the obsessions relate to the patient only, Rush calls it hypochondriasis. When relating to objects external to the patient, it is melancholia (which he renames tristimania). Amenomania, akin to paranoia is another type of partial intellectual derangement. General intellectual derangement also has three forms: mania, manicula (like mania but less severe) and manalgia (like schizophrenia).

Rush sometimes calls dementia, demence, from Pinel's *démence*, but more commonly, he uses his own term, dissociation. Rounding out the classification are derangements of specific mental "faculties", among which fatuity, or "the total absence of understanding and memory"; it "decays with the passions, in despotic countries." Other affected faculties include those of believing, dreaming, reverie and passions (love, grief, fear, etc.). He credits the ancient Roman poet, Ovid, with suggesting two remedies for the "disease" of love: getting a new mistress and dwelling upon all the bad qualities of the present mistress.

In summary, Rush's classification was roughly this,

- Intellectual derangement
    - Partial
        - Hypochondriasis
        - Tristimania
        - Amenomonia
    - General
        - Mania
        - Manicula
        - Manalgia
- Dissociation
- Derangements of specific faculties (numerous)

---

[22]Benjamin Rush, *Medical Inquiries and Observations upon the Diseases of the Mind.* Philadelphia, Kimber and Richardson (1812).

3 Mind, Brain or Both?

Both Pinel and Esquirol often wrote about the life circumstances surrounding their patients' illnesses. Yet neither man had much to say about the ultimate cause or causes. They viewed the illnesses in terms of either intellectual impairment or psychological disturbance, but did not speculate on what might be called the underlying mechanism. For others, however, the question of whether the ultimate cause lies in the mind, in the brain, or both is paramount. The debate about mind versus brain is a recurrent theme in the history of psychiatry. It began with Plato and Hippocrates, continued in the nineteenth century, and remains with us today.

A commonly held understanding of mind and brain was articulated by René Descartes in the seventeenth century. Descartes wrote not in Latin, as was customary at the time, but in the vernacular French language. He argued that *le cerveau* (the brain) is completely different from, and independent of, *l'áme* (the soul). Although Descartes did not comment specifically about so-called mental disorders, it is fair to assume that if he had, he would have characterized them as soul disorders. For Descartes, who was staunchly Catholic, it was perfectly natural for him to use the word, soul. Today, we seldom speak of souls outside of our churches and temples. But we do speak of minds, and mind and soul are related concepts, both referring to non-material entities. For many people, mental illness is *literally* an illness of the mind.

The brain's outward appearance reveals nothing of its function, and it was not until recently that its activity could be studied in a living human. Aristotle is reputed to have thought that the brain is an organ for cooling the blood. Other ancients, however, inferred a key role for the brain in sensation, movement and consciousness, most likely because they knew what happens to those functions when the brain is damaged. Building on that knowledge, certain physicians proposed brain-based theories of mental illness.

Hippocrates was the most astute of early physicians – so far as we know. Judging from the following statement, it appears that he believed mental illnesses to be brain illnesses.

Men ought to know that from nothing else but the brain come joys, delights, laughter and sports, and sorrows, griefs, despondency, and lamentations. And by this, in an especial manner, we acquire wisdom and knowledge, and see and hear, and know what are foul and what are fair, what are bad and what are good, what are sweet, and what unsavory ... And by the same organ we become mad and delirious, and fears and terrors assail us, some by night, and some by day, and dreams and untimely wanderings, and cares that are not suitable, and ignorance of present circumstances, desuetude, and unskillfulness. All these things we endure from the brain, when it is not healthy ...[23]

Much later, in 1650, Nicholas Malebranche got more specific. Writing about hallucinations, one of the hallmarks of severe mental illness, he proposed a mechanism based the properties of "animal spirits". Spirit is a curious word with many meanings. We usually think of it as a state of mind, but in other contexts, it refers to distilled alcoholic drinks. In Malebranche's time it meant, according to the Oxford English Dictionary, "One of certain subtle highly-refined substances or fluids ... supposed to permeate the blood and chief organs of the body." Galen, a Greek physician living in the time of the Roman empire, had proposed that animal spirits regulate brain activity, create mechanical forces and contract muscles. Variations on that theme were still prominent in the seventeenth century, when Nicolas Malebranche's came up with an explanation of hallucinations,

[It] sometimes happens that persons whose animal spirits are highly agitated by fasting, vigils, a high fever, or some violent passion have the internal fibers of their brain set in motion as forcefully as by external objects. Because of this, such people sense what they should only imagine, and they think they see objects before their eyes which are only in their imaginations.[24]

Animal spirits also entered into the proposal of Thomas Willis, an influential English doctor who published a book that has been described as "the most complete account of a brain-based psychiatry since the Greeks began practicing medicine."[25] Willis was a bright, curious gentleman who

---

[23]Hippocrates, *On the Sacred Disease.*

[24]Nicholas Malebranche, *The Search After Truth.* Edited and translated by T. M. Lennon and P. J. Olscamp. Cambridge, Cambridge University Press (1674, 1997).

[25]Carl Zimmer, *Soul Made Flesh: The Discovery of the Brain and how It Changed the World.* London, Free Press, 2004.

had a passion for examining human brains, usually brains "donated" by individuals who had been hung for committing crimes. In a famous incident, the body of a young woman who had been executed for infanticide was delivered to the home of a professor friend of Willis. When the men opened the coffin in preparation for the dissection, they were shocked by an unmistakable gagging sound. The woman, thought dead, was trying to breathe. Fortunately, Willis and his colleague were able to revive the woman. They lost an opportunity to dissect, but gained reputations as skilled physicians. Reputations aside, Willis was undoubtedly an accomplished anatomist. The best known of his discoveries is the eponymous Circle of Willis, a constellation of arteries at the base of the brain.

Willis was interested in mental disorders. After searching for anatomical correlates but finding none, he speculated. In his book, *The Soul of Brutes* (1683), he proposed that wayward spirits – of the kind discussed by Galen and Malebranche – cause tiny explosions in the brain. The resulting damage disorders brain pathways and produces mental disorders. It was a plausible hypothesis at the time, but incorrect.

While the foregoing summaries of early speculations weigh in favor of brain-based theories, it is difficult to gauge the degree to which they were widespread. Persons with strong religious leanings – like Descartes, who was a contemporary of Malebranche and Willis – would have favored soul-based explanations. Even in the early nineteenth century, one of the most prominent physicians in Germany held to a soul-based interpretation of mental illness.

Johann Heinroth was a contemporary of Pinel and Esquirol. He called the Frenchmen's classifications "lamentable". Heinroth was well aware of his patients' intellectual impairments and psychological disturbances, but he saw them as fundamentally caused by moral corruption. The contrast between Heinroth's perspective and that of Pinel and Esquirol can be explained, at least in part, by their different personal backgrounds. Whereas Pinel and Esquirol experienced the French Revolution first hand, Heinroth grew up in quiet Leipzig. As a child, he was cuddled by a very religious mother. According to the testimony of a contemporary biographer, "Her religious sensibility made a lasting impression on the sensitive disposition of her extremely vivacious son who quite early revealed the full extent of his sanguine character."[26] At school, Heinroth's interests oscillated between

---

[26]Quoted in Holger Steinberg, "The sin in the aetiological concept of Johann Christian August Heinroth (1773-1843)," part 1. *History of Psychiatry* 15:329-344 (2004a), p. 331.

theology and medicine. As a humanist and a Protestant, he approached mental illness with the same romantic passion that was then current among German intellectuals. His appointment as professor of "psychic therapy" at Leipzig University was the first European appointment specifically designated for psychiatric training.

Heinroth's textbook (1818) is a frustrating read due to its frequent repetitions and inconsistencies, but it is nonetheless fascinating. Heinroth wrote that "the person is more than just the mere body as well as more than the mere soul: it is the whole human being,"[27]. The body and the soul each affect the other, and both contribute to mental illness. Certain conditions, such as hallucinations and mood disorders, originate in the body and leave no mark on the soul. By contrast, the more serious and more interesting illnesses develop from disturbances of the soul.

When discussing Johann Heinroth, it is correct to translate his works using the word soul, because he clearly knew what he was doing when he wrote *Seele* (soul) rather than the alternative, *Geist* (mind). Only *Seele* was consistent with his religious orientation. He acknowledged the brain's role in supporting psychic functions, but he maintained that the corrupt soul is *primarily* responsible for mental illness. Brain lesions and bodily signs are simply *secondary* manifestations of the underlying cause. Hence came his use of the term psychosomatic, he being the first to use it.

There is no point, Heinroth wrote, in "carving up the body after its death to identify the causes for these degenerated states." Psychiatrists should "concentrate on analyzing the living individual instead of the dead torso."[28] Even if one were to find a brain correlate of mental illness, the discovery would explain nothing because it would represent only a consequence of the soul's disturbance, not its cause.

> If we ... make a detailed study of the past life of the patient, prior to the complete derangement of his psyche, we would perhaps find that the key to the organic degeneration of the brain and of the vessels lies in this life itself, in its wrong conduction, its excesses and debauches and that it is not these interdependent and interacting polarities which cause the soul's illness, but that the soul having gone astray changes the organic life.

---

[27] Quoted in H. Steinberg (2004a), p. 333.

[28] Holger Steinberg, "The sin in the aetiological concept of Johann Christian August Heinroth (1773-1843)," part 2. *History of Psychiatry* 15:437-454 (2004b). Quote on pp. 441-442.

> This change, however, was nothing but mere effect and not the
> cause as one is inclined to assume.[29]

Or, as a modern professor would caution his or her student, "correlation
does not *necessarily* reflect causation."

Although sin and evil are the root causes of insanity, predisposition and
experience are also relevant. Heinroth put it this way,

> All disturbances of the soul life originate from two elements, the
> mood of the soul and the stimulus, and since these elements are
> ever active in man without, however, invariably producing soul
> disturbances, it follows that ... the two elements must therefore
> be in a special relationship, and it is this relationship which we
> must now locate and determine.[30]

Here, again, Heinroth comes close to the modern view that heredity
("the mood of the soul") and the environment ("the stimulus") interact to
produce mental illness.

In other passages Heinroth stresses the role of human passions.

> All passion is truly a state of human disease which also attacks
> bodily life and casts it down to an extent depending on the
> strength or weakness of the passion... In accordance with the
> directions they take and with the states of mind they produce,
> passions form a very complex tissue in the human soul. For they
> are as varied as the objects of desire and fear and the forms
> of existence and possession can be. But all have in common
> that they rob the soul which panders to them of peace and
> freedom, and thus take the soul out of the sphere of higher
> consciousness... the man who is fettered by passion deceives
> himself about external objects and about himself. This illusion
> [delusion], and the consequent error, is called madness.[31]

Heinroth's psychiatry is not easily summarized, because it is a mix of religious themes, mind-body dualism and romantic notions of freedom. Working in a period of history when psychological interpretations of mental

---

[29] Johann Christian Heinroth, *Textbook of Disturbances of Mental Life; or, Disturbances
of the Soul and their Treatment*, translated by J. Schmorak. Baltimore, John Hopkins
University Press (1818, 1975), §140.

[30] J. C. Heinroth (1818, 1975), §177.

[31] J. C. Heinroth (1818, 1975), §39- 41.

illness were coming into conflict with neuroscientific interpretations, Heinroth contributed a useful intermediate position according to which mind *and* body deserve attention. Within that theoretical context, he saw the doctor's role as that of a companion, accompanying the patient as he or she tries to purify his or her soul. Although advocating this form of treatment, historical accounts suggest that Heinroth had very little first-hand experience with patients, which could explain the paucity of clinical description in his textbook.

Even if he had few occasions to actually interview and observe psychiatric patients, Heinroth devoted one-half of his textbook to diagnosis and classification or, as he called it, the "science of forms". His classification was a complex thing organized on the hierarchical principles laid down by the Swedish biologist, Carl Linnaeus. First, he classified illnesses according to whether they affected the mind, the spirit, or the will. Next, following Linnaeus's plan for plants and animals, he organized "the morbid conditions of the Psyche by the systematic subdivision into orders, genera, species, and varieties." Altogether, he named nine genera, which were further divided into thirty-six species. The classification includes the main illnesses identified by Pinel and Esquirol (mania, melancholia, dementia and idiocy), but also many new ones, among which quiet rage, silliness and timidity.

$$-//-$$

Heinroth's views notwithstanding, religious convictions, no matter how strong, do not necessarily dictate a person's understanding of insanity. Take, for example, the opinions of Benjamin Rush, an American contemporary of Heinroth. Rush was a fervent evangelist, yet he believed that mental illness is explained by strictly physical mechanisms. Writing in his textbook, he first rejected earlier suggestions that placed the cause of madness in the liver, the spleen, the intestines, or the nerves. "Lastly," he then states, "madness has been placed exclusively in the mind. I object to this opinion ... because the mind is incapable of any operations independently of impressions communicated to it though the medium of the body."[32] So, madness was not in any of the named body organs, nor in the mind, but rather, "the cause of madness is seated primarily in the blood-vessels of the brain."

Moreover, Rush believed that nearly *all* diseases are caused by constrictions of blood vessels. "There is nothing specific in these actions. They

---

[32]B. Rush (1812), p. 16.

are a part of the unity of disease, particularly of fever; of which madness is a chronic form, affecting that part of the brain which is the seat of the mind."[33] Like Descartes, therefore, Rush believed that the mind resides in a particular part of the brain. He does not say whether it is in the pineal gland, as Descartes maintained, or in some other place.

Each of the eight "reasons" that Rush offers in defense of his theory of constricted blood vessels qualifies as either anecdotal or conjectural. Nevertheless, and unfortunately, Rush's focus on blood vessels led him to advocate bloodletting as the treatment of choice for fevers generally and for mania especially, the latter being "the highest grade of general madness."

> It should be copious on the first attack of the disease. From 20 to 40 ounces of blood may be taken at once ... It will do most if the patient be bled in a standing posture. The effects of this early and copious bleeding are wonderful in calming mad people. It often prevents the necessity of using any other remedy, and sometimes it cures in a few hours.[34]

Although Rush was evidently a caring and concerned physician, what mattered most was the efficacy of treatment. In addition to bloodletting, he promoted use of the Gyrater, a device which rapidly spun the patient in the horizontal plane so as to direct blood into the brain. Moreover, to "secure obedience" prior to the implementation of these treatments, Rush recommended "certain modes of coercion", one of which was the Tranquilizer Chair, a restraining device designed to reduce sensory stimulation. And, "if all these modes of punishment should fail of their intended effects, it will be proper to resort to the fear of death."[35]

Back in Germany, opinion on the mind-brain issue became divided between two opposing views, each represented by its own informal alliance. In one camp were the *Psychiker*, or psychics, who believed that mental illness are *in* the mind. Opposing the *Psychiker* were the *Somatiker*, or somaticists, who maintained that only the body can become sick. The *Somatiker* did not deny the reality of psychological disturbance, but they argued that such problems are only the superficial symptoms of an underlying physical illness. These two loosely organized groups engaged in hot debates for many years.

---

[33]B. Rush (1812), pp. 17-18.
[34]B. Rush (1812), p. 187.
[35]B. Rush (1812), p. 182.

Elsewhere in Europe, opinions were similarly divided. In England, Henry Maudsley was the psychiatrist most listened to, perhaps because he presented himself as favoring both mental *and* brain-based points of view. Very active in many roles, Maudsley was a clinical psychiatrist as well as an entrepreneur, philosopher, philanthropist and author of numerous literary and medical works. He married the daughter of a successful alienist, then took over the operation of his father-in-law's private asylum. From the fees paid to Maudsley by wealthy families, and from additional monies earned through his forensic consultations and publications, Maudsley accumulated a large personal fortune.

He believed that madness is rooted in passion and anti-social selfishness. Masturbation drew Maudsley's special ire because, being anti-social in the extreme, it posed a high risk for mental illness. Another target was alcohol, which he said caused problems not only for the drinker but also for the drinker's progeny. It was a form of hereditary insanity. Drink led to drunkenness in the first generation, frenzied need in the second generation, hypochondria in the third and idiocy in the fourth.

Concurrent with these views, Maudsley held other opinions of a more modern nature. He wrote, for example, that "mental disorders are neither more nor less than nervous diseases in which mental symptoms predominate."[36] He, himself, was not a scientist but he urged others to study the brain. Unfortunately, as the historian Edward Shorter explains, "The Achilles' heel, or genius if one prefers, of English psychiatry was that it was all clinical medicine and little science. The English were known as superb observers, clinical investigators and examiners, but their clinical findings lacked the kind of anchor in the natural sciences at which the Germans were so gifted."[37]

Maudsley got his ideas about hereditary insanity from France, where the proposition was widely discussed and generally endorsed. It was part of a broader concept known as degeneration theory. This was not a theory specifically *about* mental illness, but it *involved* mental illness. And, while it did not speak directly to the mind-brain issue, it managed to incorporate both biological and moralistic perspectives in respect to mental disturbances. Supporters of degeneration theory believed that persons possessed of either a physical disability or a weak character pass their deviance on to a second generation. From the second, it passes to a third generation, then

---

[36]Henry Maudsley, *Body and Mind.* London, Macmillan (1870), p. 41.

[37]Edward Shorter, *A History of Psychiatry: From the Era of the Asylum to the Age of Prozac.* New York, John Wiley & Sons (1997), p. 90.

a fourth, and so on. With each successive generation, the severity of the disorder increases until finally the entire family lineage is extinguished. The primary disposing factor, the most commonly attributed initial cause, was thought to be alcoholic intoxication, and the most typical manifestation, mental illness.

The leading proponent of hereditary insanity was Benedict Morel, the medical director of an asylum in Rouen, France. The majority of Morel's patients came from rural, working class families, and the members of such families often drank excessive amounts of alcohol or smoked opium. Morel saw the drug abuse, and the general life styles of these people, as evidence of "degeneration". The full theory was published in an influential book published in 1857 under the exceptionally long title, *Traité des dégénérescences physiques, intellectuelles et morales de l'espèce humaine et des causes qui produisent ces variétés maladives* (*Treatise on the physical, intellectual and moral degeneracy of the human race and the causes of these sickly conditions*).

The actual evidence for hereditary degeneration was weak, and the mechanisms proposed for its transmission from generation to generation were fuzzy. Nevertheless, the theory satisfied the need for a scientific explanation of mental disorder. Moreover, its hint of biological plausibility scored big in France, where biological causes for mental illness were favored over psychological causes. Thus, degeneration became popular as a way of explaining insanity.

Degeneration theory met a more mixed reception In Germany. Wilhelm Griesinger, a sage psychiatrist with generally progressive opinions (discussed below), endorsed the idea. In the widely read second edition of his 1861 textbook, Griesinger wrote,

> The disposition (to hereditary degeneration) may disappear by constantly renewing the blood by marriage with perfectly healthy families; it is increased and developed to the most degenerate forms by further intermarriages, by drunkenness of fathers, et cetera ... The deterioration of a whole race, as well as the special degeneration of a particular patient generally occurs gradually and progressively ... It appears ... that hereditary influence may be highly and quickly increased by drunkenness, by disease, and in short, by various intercurrent disorders of the parents at the time of procreation.[38]

---

[38] Quoted in W. F. Bynum, "Alcoholism and degeneration in 19th century European medicine and psychiatry," *British Journal of Addiction* 79: 59-70 (1984), p. 61.

Another ardent supporter of degeneration was Richard Krafft-Ebing, the Austrian whose *Zwangvorstellung* had led to so much confusion over the naming of obsessive disorders. In addressing the problems of children born of alcoholic parents, he wrote,

> They come into the world as idiots, with hydrocephalous [severely enlarged heads] or neurotic-convulsive constitutions and perish in early years of convulsions. In those who survive, epilepsy, hysteria, mental diseases, and weakness, and exactly the severest forms of mental impairment are developed out the morbid constitution of the nerve-centers.

When Krafft-Ebing came to describing the hereditary consequences of alcoholism, the downward spiral resembled the warnings issued earlier by Morel and Maudsley.

> First generation: Moral depravity, alcoholic excess.
>
> Second generation: Drink mania, attacks of insanity, general paralysis.
>
> Third generation: Hypochondria, melancholia, apathy, and tendencies to murder.
>
> Fourth generation: Imbecility, idiocy, and extinction of family.[39]

Krafft-Ebing later became famous for his book, *Psychopathia Sexualis*, the essence of which is well summarized by Edward Shorter,

> By the time [he wrote this book], Krafft-Ebing was seeing degeneration literally under the bed. The onanists [masturbators], homosexuals, and premature ejaculators who paraded through its pages ... were virtually without exception stamped as 'degenerates'. The book remains a classic example of psychiatry run off the rails ...[40]

In contrast to Griesinger and Krafft-Ebing, Emil Kraepelin and Sigmund Freud had their doubts about degeneration, and neither promoted it as an explanation for mental illness. They accepted that heredity plays a role in

---

[39]Both quotations from Axel Gustafson, *The Foundations of Death: A Study of the Drink-Question*. Boston, Ginn Heath (1885), pp. 178-179.
[40]E. Shorter (1997), p. 96.

causing certain psychiatric conditions, but not a dominant part as claimed by the proponents of degeneration theory. Their skepticism contributed to declining support for the theory. Also weighing in against degeneration theory was the re-examination of some data that had supposedly proved it, and the biological implausibility of acquired characteristics being inherited. The theory gradually faded away, and by the end of the nineteenth century, it had almost entirely disappeared.

Looking back, we can see that degeneration theory served to deflect public opinion from the overcrowded asylums where patients languished without hope. It also fed a growing distaste for the disadvantaged, disfigured and deviant members of society. The theory's dark, racial overtones grew from a peculiar Darwinian view of human history which saw the human species headed downward toward an ignominious end. Because it was a way of thinking that led to eugenics and Nazi policies of racial purification, it is easy to dismiss degeneration theory as scientifically misguided and morally questionable. But we still believe that heredity plays a role in the genesis of mental illness, and we still grapple, as did nineteenth century psychiatrists, with understanding precisely what that role is.

Degeneration theory skirted, but did not deeply engage the mind-brain issue. It came closest when emphasizing hereditary predispositions. Before the mid-1800s, heredity was a vague concept largely synonymous with the inheritance of wealth and social standing. It had little or no connection to physiology, anatomy, or any other biological phenomenon. That view was changing, however, at the same time as degeneration theory was taking root. People started thinking of hereditary transmission in terms of biological reproduction. So, some credit is due degeneration theory for drawing attention to the body as a possible factor in mental illness, even if the inference was weak and the hypothetical mechanism flawed.

Loose thinking about mind-brain relations led some psychiatrists into odd places. That happened to David Skae, a physician at the Royal Edinburgh Asylum. Publishing in the *Journal of Mental Science*, he offered readers a classification of mental illnesses that was both "rational and practical." He believed that all insanities either originate in the body or are expressed in the body. Different illnesses are associated with different body parts or different bodily functions. Thus, Skae's classification included disorders with such names such mania of masturbation, mania of pregnancy, sunstroke mania and metastatic mania. Oddly, because he had a peculiar concept of the mind as a physical entity, he even characterized idiocy and senility as body-based mental illnesses. Skae defended his classification

with the statement, "It has this especial merit at least, that it ever keeps
before us the all-important principle that insanity is a disease of the *body*,
whether it be of some remote organ sympathetically acting on the mind, or
of the material organ of the mind itself [italics original]."[41] Whatever that
means.

[41]David Skae, "A rational and practical classification of insanity." *Journal of Mental
Science* IX (47): 309-319 (1863).

4 A New Vision for Psychiatry

The first half of the nineteenth century saw the elimination, or at least the lessening, of harsh practices in hospitals and asylums, but otherwise little had changed on the ground. The doctors had no effective treatments, and the patients little comfort. Although headway had been made in cutting mental illness at its joints, the fundamental nature of mental disorder was still being debated at mid-century, with moral interpretations vying with biological interpretations, and psychological causes weighing in against neurological causes. Degeneration theory seemed, at first, to provide answers, but its light was fading. Meanwhile, the *Somatiker* battled the *Psychiker*, hoping to score a knockout with solid evidence of neurological abnormalities. Thus, while the first half of the nineteenth century occasioned a general uptick of interest in psychiatry, at mid-century the field as a whole looked more or less as it had fifty years earlier.

In Germany at this time, psychiatric patients were housed in about one hundred different institutions. Most were located in rural areas and known as asylums. They had been placed in the countryside because rural lands were cheap, and the sparsely populated areas provided a degree of protection for patients who might otherwise be subjected to public scorn. Apart from these benefits, asylum doctors believed that it was good for patients to be in the countryside, because it removed them from the negative influences of family, friends and urban stresses.

The German asylums, like those elsewhere in Europe, were still horrible places. Patients lived in overcrowded, barrack-like buildings where relief came only from sedation and baths. A minority of patients got better and were released, but the majority faced long periods of confinement. Patients suffering from acute mental breakdowns where frequently mixed with patients lost in incurable dementias. Unruly patients were routinely restrained, and sometimes physically punished.

Gradually, madness came to be seen not just as a social problem, but also as a medical problem. Accordingly, it was thought desirable to place some institutions for the insane in cities, where doctors could link up with the local university. These urban institutions were generally smaller than their rural cousins. They were known as "clinics" or "hospitals", and they were intended primarily for short-term patient care.

Just as the daily lives of patients were beginning to improve, a serious problem arose in the asylums. Coming unannounced and unexplained, a rising tide of admissions swamped the facilities. Directors and administrators struggled to cope with the increasing numbers, details of which scholars later recovered. In Germany, in 1852, the ratio of asylum patients to ordinary citizens was one in 5,300; by 1911 that ratio had risen to one in five hundred. England also saw an astonishing rate of increase in its patient population. Whereas the average English asylum held 116 patients in 1827, that number had reached 1,072 by 1910. Similarly in the United States, the average number of patients per asylum was 57 in 1820, but 473 in 1870. Remarkably, patient numbers at individual asylums increased even though there were more asylums operating than ever before. At the beginning of the century, there were few asylums in any European country, but by the end of the century, France had 108 asylums and the German-speaking countries had 402.[42]

Why admissions increased so sharply, is not completely understood. Historians point to changing social attitudes as one factor. They cite a growing trend toward casting out deviant citizens, whether mentally ill or poor or eccentric. Thus, many persons with no actual mental illness wound up in asylums. At the same time, some poorhouses and prisons that had previously housed mentally ill persons, stopped doing so, thus forcing nearly all psychiatric patients into those same asylums. It is also possible that there was an increase in the incidence of mental illness. Statistical evidence suggests rising rates for several diagnostic types, specifically progressive paralysis, delirium tremor (from alcoholism) and schizophrenia. If mental illness did, in fact, become more common, it would have been due to social factors, gene mutations, or possibly both. Regardless of the cause or causes of the overcrowding, it put the brakes on all substantial reforms. Moreover, even custodial care suffered a setback due to pressed infrastructures and overwhelmed work forces.

In the midst of all of this, a twenty-eight year old German doctor with less than six years of practice – mostly in general medicine – published a searing criticism of mental asylums. The author was Wilhelm Griesinger. He was born in Stuttgart and educated at universities in Tübingen and Zurich. He was a very smart man, and he was calling for a new way of doing psychiatry.

---

[42]Data from Shorter (1997), pp. 34, 46-48.

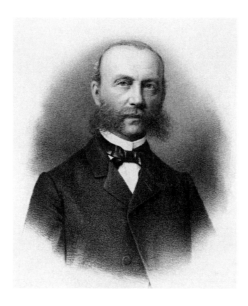

Figure 3: Wilhelm Griesinger.

Griesinger launched his attack in 1845, at a time when European psychiatry was squarely centered on the asylum. Alienist physicians, mostly employed by the state, were expected to provide clean, safe accommodations for patients, but little else. Some went further, of course, striving for a therapeutic community or experimenting with forms of moral therapy, but the measures were largely ineffective. On the whole, misery and pessimism prevailed in the overcrowded asylums.

Eric Engstrom, an authority on nineteenth century German asylums, has brought to light another aspect of the alienists' work: their reliance on a peculiar managerial strategy.

> Alienists emphasized the practical orientation of their research and juxtaposed it to [contrasted it with] the theoretical constructions and cerebral hypotheses of schoolmen [university professors]. The focal point of their work was the construction and maintenance of a therapeutic environment within an institutional setting. They spent an enormous amount of time working up, implementing, and fine-tuning institutional rules governing space, time, movement, diet, discipline, and hygiene... Alienists were in many senses therapeutic choreographers for whom the

asylum's efficient organization and their own medical skills comprised the dramaturgical stuff of therapeutic practice.[43]

In other words, the alienists believed that they could soften the blows of mental illness by putting on a convincing show of medical authority and knowhow.

For Griesinger, this was not nearly enough. He blasted institutional psychiatry for its use of mechanical restraints, its empty science, and its phony standard of cures. He thought German society was capable of something better, a new kind of psychiatry that would be based on the primacy of neurological science. Here is the first paragraph of his textbook,

> Insanity itself, an anomalous condition of the faculties of knowledge and of will, is only a symptom; our classification of the group of mental diseases proceeds upon the symptomatological method, and by such a method, and by such a method alone can any classification be effected. The first step towards a knowledge of the symptoms is their locality – to which organ do the indications of the disease belong? What organ must necessarily and invariably be diseased where there is madness? ... Physiological and pathological facts show us that this organ can only be the brain; we therefore primarily, and in every case of mental disease, recognize a morbid action of that organ.[44]

In another passage, Griesinger provided a concise statement of where psychiatry should be headed. It is remarkable, not only because it turned out to be an accurate prediction of what psychiatry later became, but also for its pointed reference to the mind-brain issue.

> Psychiatry has undergone a transformation in its relationship to the rest of medicine. This transformation rests principally on the realization that patients with so-called mental illnesses are really individuals with illnesses of the nerves and brain. [Psychiatry must therefore] emerge from its closed-off status as a guild and become an integral part of general medicine accessible to all medical circles.[45]

---

[43]Eric J. Engstrom, *Clinical Psychiatry in Imperial Germany: A History of Psychiatric Practice*. Ithaca, Cornell University Press (2003), pp. 88-89.

[44]Wilhelm Griesinger, *Mental Pathology and Therapeutics*, translated by C. L. Robertson and J. Rutherford. London, The New Sydenham Society (1861, 1867), p. 1.

[45]Wilhelm Griesinger, *Archiv für Psychiatrie und Nervenkrankheiten* (1868), p. 3.

The key sentence in the above passage is often quoted inaccurately. Because he wrote, " ... dass die sogenannten 'Geisteskranken' hirn- und nervenkranke Individuen sind," the passage should translate as, "patients with so-called mental illnesses are really individuals with illnesses of the nerves and brain." More commonly, it is rendered as "mental illnesses are brain illnesses." The simplification distorts the meaning and undermines the intent. The comment was directed toward the *Somatiker*, who had long argued for a biological approach to mental illness. They, however, had not put any special emphasis on the brain, suggesting instead that many different bodily defects could create conditions for mental illness (recall David Skae's classification). Griesinger, by contrast, is suggesting here that mental illnesses are *exclusively* illnesses of the brain. Elsewhere, he stressed that the proposition, while probably true, had not yet been proven. He himself was neither an anatomist nor a physiologist. He called upon those who were practicing scientists to uncover definitive proof, by finding evidence of brain pathologies.

Griesinger was in the right place at the right time. Following the success of the industrial revolution, scientific inquiry had found new purposes and new tools. It had moved from its former home among philosophers to a new base occupied by observers and experimenters. The transformation began in England, then spread quickly to Germany and the rest of Europe. Its forerunners were Michael Faraday and James Clerk Maxwell (electromagnetism), Charles Lyell (geology) and Charles Darwin (biology).

It is not widely known that Darwin was interested in mental illness, but he wrote about it in his book, *Expression of the Emotions* (1872). His main goal in that book was to persuade readers that human expressions are "descended with modification" from our animal ancestors. To support the argument, Darwin studied and reported on the faces of insane people. According to the Darwinian scholar Janet Browne, he did so because,

> he believed their emotions were uncontrolled and intense, and that, rather like children, their faces would display their feelings in a pure, uncomplicated way, ideal for a scientific survey of expressions. The passions would be more strongly accentuated and easier to identify; emotions less complex than in the sane.[46]

Darwin obtained dozens of photographs of insane patients and included a few in his book. While some physiognomists claimed that they could diag-

---

[46] Janet Browne, " Darwin and the face of madness," in *The Anatomy of Madness*, vol. 1, eds. W.F. Bynum, R. Porter, and M. Shepherd. London, Tavistock (1985), p. 153.

nose a specific mental illness by examining the patient's facial expressions, Darwin did not see discrete "species" of madness – only generic emotions such as distress, rage, fear and sorrow. Overall, the impact of Darwin's writings on psychiatry was small. More influential, was the fact that Darwin had built his whole theory of evolution on detailed, unbiased observations. It was the very method that Griesinger was urging upon the new breed of psychiatrists.

Griesinger's views were shaped by the work of a number of scientists who happened also to be doctors (but not psychiatrists). Carl von Rokitansky, for example, was a Viennese pathologist who personally performed over 30,000 autopsies. Griesinger heard his call for objective methods in the medical sciences, and he endorsed it. Griesinger was also influenced by the Parisian physiologist, François Magendie, in whose laboratory Griesinger spent several months. Magendie showed him how nervous messages travel from the brain to the spinal cord and then out from the spinal cord into peripheral nerves. From these observations, Griesinger developed a theory of mental reflexes, which I describe below. It was Johannes Müller, however, who made the biggest impression on the young Griesinger.

Müller was a licensed physician in Berlin, but he did not practice medicine. He was, instead, a research scientist who investigated an impressive range of topics using the tools of microscopy, comparative anatomy and neurophysiology. From his neurophysiological experiments, he developed a theory of "specific nerve energies", according to which each of the sensory nerves imparts a special flavor to its electrical messages. The brain then "reads" or "interprets" the specific energies, thus yielding the unique subjective experiences of sight, hearing, taste, et cetera. The idea was creative, and plausible at the time, but incorrect. Apart from laboratory work, Müller was fascinated by a group of rare marine animals, which he attempted to classify in the manner of Darwin. Griesinger took from Müller a love of science and a deep respect for careful observation. He also learned that it is not enough to simply gather facts – one needs to reflect upon those facts and build theories based on them. This, instead of speculation.

And lastly, Griesinger admired the work of Rudolf Virchow. A pupil of Müller, Virchow was likewise a polymath. He was active as a physician, anthropologist, pathologist, prehistorian, biologist, writer, editor and politician. Not just active, but talented too. His pioneering experiments revealed the vital importance of biological cells in health and disease.

Griesinger was inspired by all the science mentioned above, but the only science that he himself did was of the armchair variety. An example of his scientific thinking was his neurological theory of mental illness. From his familiarity with the physiological investigations of François Magendie and Johannes Müller, he knew that sensory signals enter the spinal cord and motor signals (commanding actions) go out from it. Thus, the spinal cord contains simple nervous circuits that mediate the unconscious behaviors of animals and certain rudimentary behaviors in humans. Extrapolating from these facts, and assuming that conscious thoughts and goals are types of higher-order reflexes, he concluded that the brain must be host to what he called "mental reflexes". Modelled on spinal reflexes, Griesinger's mental reflexes connected one thought to another. He believed, in this context, that any sort of extreme physiological activity – involving either too much neural excitation or too little excitation – would adversely affect mental functions, and that if such extreme states of activity persisted, they would result in psychiatric illness. Griesinger' theory was clever and based on the latest scientific knowledge. Its only problem? It was untestable and hence speculative, the very sort of theory that he would have denounced had it come from anyone else.

Although Griesinger is remembered as a pioneer of modern psychiatry, he saw himself first and foremost as a doctor of internal medicine, the field in which he trained and in which he spent the bulk of his career. In his early years, he held positions as either physician or professor – or both simultaneously – at half a dozen different institutions in as many locations, including one in Egypt where he acted as the personal physician to the Viceroy of Cairo. He wrote a big book on Egyptian public health, established a professional journal devoted to general medicine, and published numerous articles on pathology and internal medicine. His seminal contributions to psychiatry came later.

In 1860, Griesinger moved to Zurich, where he had studied medicine many years earlier. He was made head of the department of internal medicine and director of a run-down mental asylum. He must have spent much of the first year revising his psychiatric textbook – originally published in 1845 – because the second edition was hailed as groundbreaking when it appeared in 1861, just one year after his arrival in Zurich.

Griesinger's ideas on psychiatry became so widely disseminated, and so much admired, that he was next appointed professor of psychiatry in Berlin. It was a prestigious position that came with two directorships. One was at the clinic for "ordinary nervous diseases", the other at the clinic for "ner-

vous diseases with a primary psychiatric presentation." Griesinger switched
his teaching duties from one clinic to the other in alternating semesters.

There was talk of merging the two clinics, but that did not happen,
primarily because of Griesinger's insistence that psychiatry and neurology
remain as separate medical fields. While he believed that all mental illnesses
are brain illnesses, he did not believe that every brain illness is necessarily
a psychiatric illness. He explained it this way,

> As insanity is only a complication of symptoms of various mor-
> bid states of the brain, the question might be asked, whether
> its special study apart from that of the other diseases of the
> brain can be justified, or whether mental pathology should not
> always accompany cerebral pathology. But, although at some
> more distant period this may perhaps be looked for, any at-
> tempt at such a combination would at present be premature
> and quite impractical.[47]

When it came to the relationship between mind and brain, Griesinger
was a philosophical materialist. He thought of the brain as a special kind
of machine. Nevertheless, he did not refrain from writing of "purposes"
and "aims", both of which, he assumed, were involved in the operation
of mental reflexes. Moreover, he did not deny the existence of souls. He
offered these deep thoughts in regard to the soul,

> While we are forced by facts to refer understanding and will to
> the brain, still, nothing can be assumed as to the relation exist-
> ing between these mental acts and the brain, the relation of soul
> to material. From an empirical point of view the unity of soul
> and body is indeed a fact primarily to be maintained, and the
> *a priori* investigation of the possibility of soul apart from body,
> of a bodiless soul, must be entirely dismissed ... How a material
> physical act in the nerve fibers or cells can be converted into an
> idea, an act of consciousness, is absolutely incomprehensible ...
> [I]t is scientifically admissible ... to consider the understanding
> and the will as the function, the special energy, of the brain,
> just as transmission and reflex action are considered the special
> function of the nerves and spinal cord, and to consider the soul
> primarily and pre-eminently as the sum of all cerebral states.[48]

---

[47]W. Griesinger (1861, 1867), p. 9.
[48]W. Griesinger (1861, 1867), pp. 3-4.

If one were to substitute the word "mind" for Griesinger's "soul", the statement quoted above could pass as a commentary written by a twenty-first century neuroscientist or philosopher.

Psychiatry was not included in the state medical examination, but it was part of the medical curriculum in Berlin. Students wishing to practice psychiatry were instructed in psychology, neuroanatomy and related academic subjects, while the old institutional psychiatry – asylum psychiatry – was largely ignored. Hearing of this, the asylum doctors (alienists) grew understandably upset. "They found themselves at once reiterating psychiatry's status as a legitimate branch of medicine, while at the same time insisting that psychiatric science required asylum-based knowledge and wholly different diagnostic skills from those learned at the university."[49] Brushing aside the alienists' insistence on "asylum-based knowledge", the medical specialty of psychiatry moved ahead along the road cleared by Griesinger.

Griesinger died in 1868, just three years after taking charge at the *Charité*, and just seven years after publishing his major work. With psychiatry now recognized as a legitimate medical discipline, mental illness started to be researched just like any other medical condition, and universities started appointing medical school professors as much on their qualifications in research as on their clinical experience. Professors of psychiatry were expected to have expertise in heredity, brain anatomy and physiology. The University of Berlin and its associated hospital, the *Charité*, led in this regard, but schools elsewhere in Europe quickly followed suit. The result was a new intellectual framework for understanding mental illness. It was an exciting time, especially in Germany, and especially for men.

One man strongly affected by Griesinger's vision was Carl Wernicke, a talented neurologist who worked briefly at Griesinger's *Charité*. Addressing the annual meeting of the prestigious *Gesellschaft Deutscher Naturforscher und Ärzte* (Society of German Scientists and Physicians) twelve years after Griesinger's death, Wernicke's words echoed Griesinger's progressive vision of basic research at the service of psychiatry. And he went further, suggesting that psychiatrists might apply their scientific knowledge toward an equally worthy objective. Mental illnesses, he said, provide "natural experiments" that can elucidate *normal* brain functions. It was a brilliant insight and fully in line with Griesinger's teachings.

---

[49]E. J. Engstrom (2003), pp. 68-69.

Let us confidently distinguish psychiatry's practical and scientific goals! As laudable as it is for psychiatric practitioners to fulfill their difficult therapeutic calling, psychiatry is also a branch of the natural sciences. As such, it has tasks to perform which are every bit as worthy as other great tasks of natural science. For it must observe and explain not only deviations from healthy mental life. It must also derive from these deviations useful information which the diseases, as natural experiments, tend to have for knowledge of the normal function of an organ. Only modern physiology of the brain will enable us to perform this task.[50]

---

[50]Quoted in E. J. Engstrom (2003), p. 101.

5 Bernhard Gudden at the Upper Bavarian District Mental Hospital

Bernhard Gudden was another German psychiatrist influenced by Wilhelm Griesinger's progressive ideas. He understood that psychiatry was headed in a new direction. It was going to a place where patients would be treated respectfully and the root causes of their disorders would be studied scientifically. Four years after Griesinger's death, Gudden moved from Zurich to Munich, where he put into practice many of the reforms urged by Griesinger. He made no major discoveries or authored any groundbreaking books, but he nurtured the new psychiatry by means of his teaching, hospital administration and anatomical research. Gudden's professional activities typified the new psychiatry. They also demonstrated its recently acquired power and prestige.

Gudden became the director of Munich's mental hospital in 1872, just one year after the birth of the German nation. Prior to that time, Germany comprised a collection of independent states linked by a common language and, in many respects, common histories. Unification came about after several of those states fought and won the Franco-Prussian War. That war was started by two powerful men harboring incompatible ambitions. Otto von Bismarck was a Prussian statesman intent on creating a united German nation under Prussian control, while Napoleon III (Charles-Louis Napoleon Bonaparte) wanted to regain some of the prestige lost by his country in earlier military and diplomatic adventures. Prussia's army was stronger than France's, and the fate of the French side became sealed once four other German states joined Prussia in the battle. The Germans laid siege to Paris and captured Napoleon. Then, just prior to France's capitulation, the German nation – or German empire (*Deutsches Reich*) – was born. Wilhelm I became the Kaiser, or king, and Otto von Bismarck, the all-important chancellor. Germany was at last a united country, proud and strong. Possessed of a large, well-equipped military and political acumen, it confidently engaged in European politics and acquired its first colonies.

The empire comprised twenty-seven states, of which Prussia was by far the largest. Bavaria was the second largest state, but also a kingdom. The king of Bavaria was Ludwig II. He was preceded by his father, Maximillian II, who was a delft politician and a popular leader. Maximillian had spent freely on infrastructure, especially in Munich, the capital city. By contrast, Ludwig II disliked politics and did little to support public institutions. He put his energies – and considerable monies – into building castles and sponsoring theater performances. Nonetheless, Bavaria grew and prospered in the early years of the German Empire. The population of Munich grew from about 100,000 in 1852 to about 250,000 in 1883.

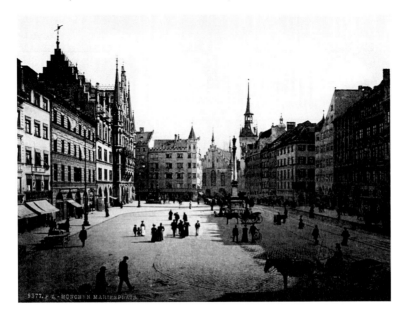

Figure 4: Marienplatz, Munich, about 1890. [Munich Municipal Archives]

In the spring of 1872, Bernhard Gudden (later, Bernhard von Gudden, thanks to his gentrification) was looking for a new job. At the time, he was working two good jobs in a lovely city, but still he wanted to move. One job was director of the Cantonal Psychiatric Clinic in southeastern Zurich, called the Burgholzli for the hill upon which it rested. His other job was professor of psychiatry at the University of Zurich. Gudden, his wife and their nine children were happy in Zurich. Their accommodations were comfortable, the schools good and Gudden's income more than adequate. The clinic building had just recently been constructed according to an architectural plan designed by Wilhelm Griesinger. The problem was, Gudden and the hospital's chief administrator did not get along. When Gudden heard that the director of the Upper Bavarian District Mental Hospital had died, he saw an opportunity. He had previously worked at a mental asylum in Bavaria, so he was familiar with the system. There was also the lure of Munich. The large, bustling city was now part of the German Empire. As such, it was fully capable of providing the director of its mental hospital with all the resources that he might need or want.

Gudden was well qualified for the job in Munich. Born in the town of Cleves in the Prussian province of Rhineland, he was the third of seven sons in a middle class family. He studied philosophy at the University of Bonn for a short while, but then switched to medicine. In those days, medical students often trained at multiple schools. Gudden studied in Bonn, Halle and Berlin. His first job was at a mental asylum in Siegburg, near Bonn, where he worked as an assistant to the head doctor and married the boss's granddaughter. Next, he was appointed director of the District Mental Hospital at Werneck in northeastern Bavaria, and after that, director at the Burgholzli clinic in Zurich. He was a heavy-set man with a large, cube-shaped head and a bushy beard. Professional in attitude and demeanor, he was highly cultured and able to chat knowledgeably about literature, music and theatre. Moreover, he had a sense of humor.

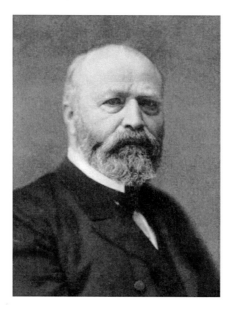

Figure 5: Bernhard Gudden, c. 1870.

It was expected that the director of the Munich hospital would also be the professor of psychiatry at the local university, as was the arrangement in Zurich. However, the process of hiring for the two positions was complicated, because the Ministry of the Interior for Church and School Affairs was responsible for the hospital, while the *Ludwig-Maximilians-Universität* was responsible for choosing its professors. As competitions for the two positions developed, communications between the ministry and the university broke down. Consequently, just as Gudden received notice from the minister that he had been appointed director of the hospital, he learned from other sources that the university was not on board. The university was expecting that a different man, not Gudden, would be appointed director, so it appointed *that* person as its professor of psychiatry. Gudden refused to accept the directorship without the professorship. Caught in a difficult situation, partly of its own making, the university relented. It gave Gudden's competitor an *honorary* professorship, and Gudden got an ordinary professorship to go along with his directorship.

The place where Gudden came to work was called the *Oberbayerische Kreisirrenanstalt*. A literal translation of *Kreisirrenanstalt* yields "district mental institution", but English-speaking authors generally refer to the Munich establishment as either the Upper Bavarian District Mental *Asylum* or the Upper Bavarian District Mental *Hospital*. The ambiguity is significant, because in reality the institution was an asylum when Gudden took charge, but a hospital at the time of his premature death. I will call it a hospital.

Munich's mental hospital was one of the largest in all the German-speaking lands, but it was otherwise typical. It was situated in an agricultural area southeast of the city, about one mile from the Isar River and two miles from the city center. With a location that partook of both rural and urban qualities, and with a mandate that was both custodial and instructional, it was perched on the cusp of modernity. The building itself was an austere looking, brown sandstone structure standing three stories tall. A line of closely spaced windows stretched monotonously from one end of the long building to the other, interrupted only by an ornamental central entrance. The symmetrical architectural plan was designed to accommodate male and female patients in separate areas. Built in 1859, the hospital was designed to house 280 patients, but it was holding about 500 when Gudden arrived.

The main function of the hospital was, of course, to accommodate and care for its patients. Nevertheless, a large space was reserved for neuroanatomical research. Gudden was convinced that studies of the brain were absolutely necessary for the advancement of psychiatry, and he evi-

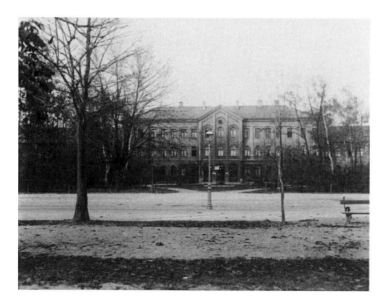

Figure 6: Upper Bavarian District Mental Hospital, 1907.

dently enjoyed the hands-on activity, because he worked in the laboratory whenever free of other obligations. He started doing research many years earlier, while working at an asylum in the town of Werneck. Some of the patients had damaged earlobes – probably from beatings – and Gudden decided to examine their wounds. Thrilled by the sight of human tissues viewed under a microscope, he redirected his curiosity from the ear to the brain, and from that point onward, he was hooked. His infectious enthusiasm for neuroanatomy led many students and co-workers to lend their hands in the laboratory, Emil Kraepelin and Franz Nissl among them.

Gudden was able to work in the laboratory as much as he did because he had installed a well-defined hierarchy of command and a finely tuned system of delegation. Gudden was the absolute boss. His immediate assistants were young psychiatrists who handled most of the patient work. They, in turn, were supported by nurses (both male and female) and students. The unskilled laborers took care of everything else. Gudden was stern with his subordinates – as was customary for persons in positions of authority – but relaxed with professional colleagues. He established numerous rules and regulations. For example, patients were allowed no more than three and one-half liters of beer per day (yes 3.5 liters!), unless the patient's family had "arranged" for more.

The patient population comprised a diverse group of individuals suffering from a numbing variety of physical and mental disorders. They came either from Munich itself or from nearby villages, and most were persons of modest means. If the family had money, the sick person was sent not to Gudden's publically funded hospital, but to a private asylum where conditions were marginally better. The patients seldom changed their clothing, and few paid much attention to personal hygiene. From day to day, there was little for them to do. Some patients wandered silently about, while others sat and talked – often to themselves. It was not uncommon to encounter a patient rocking back and forth, or otherwise moving his or her limbs in repetitive, stereotyped patterns. Loud shouts were occasionally heard, as was raucous laughter and sobbing. Contrastingly, there were patients who never uttered a sound. The air contained a heavy mix of tobacco smoke, body odors, vomit and the pungent scent of choral hydrate, which was the drug of choice for calming and sedating patients.

Leading off from the main corridor of Gudden's hospital were five rooms, each with about thirty beds. These rooms were for sleeping, primarily at night, but also during the day for patients who had been given a sedative. Other patients, sedated or not, lay on floors throughout the hospital. Apart from medicated sedation, the only other treatments – if they may be called that – were bed rests and baths (hydrotherapy). Bed rests were ordinarily combined with sedation. The numbing effect of the drug rendered the patient more manageable, while the tranquility of the bed quieted his or her inner turmoil. In this way, patients would sometimes remain in the sleeping room for days on end.

Baths, like bed rests, had long been used throughout continental Europe as well as in Great Britain and North America. Some practitioners preferred them hot, others cold and sudden. After first learning about baths while working as an assistant physician in the Munich hospital, Emil Kraepelin later employed them frequently. He wrote about the Munich experience in his *Memoirs*, stating that baths were sometimes used "for weeks and months", but it is unclear whether he was referring to continuous or intermittent submersion. In describing one particular case, however, his meaning was unambiguous, "Once, I left a very agitated patient in the bath for three days, because it was too great a risk to put her into the isolation room and she could not be kept in bed."[51]

Despite the liberal use of sedatives, bed rests and baths, there were always patients whose troublesome, even violent, behaviors presented a dan-

---

[51]Emil Kraepelin, *Memoirs*. Berlin, Springer-Verlag (1987), p. 40.

ger to themselves and others. Verbal arguments, assaults and fights were commonplace. Kraepelin recalled what he saw,

> There were a great number of fights, the smashing of windows or crockery. I often had to bandage or sew the wounds caused by these fights. In those days, the wrong-doers were punished by stopping the small amounts of beer allowed [3.5 liters per day!]. This only led to increased outbreaks of abusive language and attacks on the doctor.[52]

Hospital staff dealt with unruly patients using a variety of measures. Punishments, for example, went beyond the denial of beer to include denials of exercise, recreation and family visits. Physical restraining devices, such as straight-jackets, iron hand-cuffs, leg-cuffs and chains, were also employed. In one instance, according to Kraepelin, a doctor accidently chained himself while trying to secure the legs of a patient. Sometimes patients were bound to special chairs. And, sadly, some of the staff beat disobedient patients.

Self-mutilation was another big concern. Psychotic patients heard voices from inside their heads urging them to commit violent acts, and sometimes they directed those acts towards themselves. Likewise, depressed patients vented their emotions upon their own bodies. Men banged their heads against walls until blood flowed from their foreheads. Patients scratched themselves relentlessly, gnawed at their fingers and pulled out their hair. Others injured themselves with knives, nails, or scissors, leaving wounds that became infected. To prevent or minimize these actions, the hospital staff had closets full of protective devices. There were leather muffs, leather mitts and long leather sleeves – all designed to be tear-proof. A type of straight-jacket was also used. It was a large gown that closed with screws instead of buttons.

The most dangerous patients were put in barren, locked chambers known as isolation rooms. A patient could be kept in an isolation room for months or even years. Sometimes problems arose. In one such episode, as recalled by Kraepelin, a scream was heard near one of the isolation rooms. Rushing to the scene, Kraepelin realized that a colleague and two male nurses were locked inside. A burly patient had freed himself, then forced the others into the room before securing the lock. When Kraepelin attempted to open the locked door, the patient leapt out, grabbed Kraepelin, and brought him to the ground. Kraepelin was wearing a heavy fur coat, so he could not easily

---

[52]E. Kraepelin (1987), p. 11.

resist. The patient grabbed Kraepelin's throat and started to squeeze, but just then a nearby patient heard the shouting and came to the rescue, freeing Kraepelin and subduing the attacker.

Gudden knew of these events and he disapproved of them. They were troublesome, but not unique to the Munich hospital. In England, an alienist by the name of John Conolly had earlier encountered similar situations. In the 1840s, he began advocating for reforms that would reduce the need for harsh measures such as those described above. He asserted that "the management of a large asylum is not only practicable without the application of bodily coercion to the patient, but ... after the total disuse of such a method of control, the whole character of the asylum undergoes a gradual and beneficial change." Conolly's book, *Treatment of the Insane without Mechanical Restraints* (1856) caused quite a stir, and as a result, several English asylums implemented his policy of "no-restraint". It proved so successful at the Hanwell County Lunatic Asylum in Middlesex that *The Times* lauded it as "one of the greatest works that the dictates of the human mind could suggest."[53]

Thus, long before coming to Munich, Gudden had read of no restraint. It was the kind of patient care that he hoped to adopt. As director of the asylum in Werneck, he had written in one of his daily reports, "But we regard as even more important than the elimination of mechanical force, the ... strengthening of even the smallest vestiges of freedom of the mind and the rejection of every form of spiritual oppression."[54] Later in Zurich, Gudden took steps – evidently incomplete – towards eliminating chains and unlocking rooms.

Thus, after tolerating all sorts of physical restraints during the first seven years of his directorship in Munich, Gudden acted decisively to stop it. He did so by publishing a notice that was addressed to the nurses, but intended for the entire staff. Widely distributed within the hospital and later elsewhere, the document formalized the modernization of patient care within psychiatric institutions.

    1. Nursing is a difficult and responsible profession. Those who dedicate themselves to this profession, must be sympathetic

---

[53] Andrew Scull, " A Victorian alienist: John Conolly," in *The Anatomy of Madness*, vol. 1., eds. W.F. Bynum, R. Porter, and M. Shepherd. London, Tavistock (1985), pp. 103-150. Quotes on pp. 121, 123.

[54] Quoted in A. Danek, W. Gudden, and H. Distel, "The dream king's psychiatrist Bernhard von Gudden (1824-1886)," *Archives of Neurology* 46: 1349-1353 (1989), p. 1349.

towards the suffering of fellow human beings, and must rid themselves of all prejudice in respect of the mentally ill.

2. No one is to blame for becoming ill and similarly, even the best, quietest and most sensible people can become mentally ill. No one is immune to becoming mentally ill. Mental disease is a disease of the brain and the brain, like all other organs, can be damaged in its activity and capacity for the most varying reasons.

3. In most cases mental diseases eliminate one's self-control. No mentally ill person can be blamed for what he does or does not do. Even if he seems to be particularly malicious and annoys and tortures those who surround him in what seems to be an intentional manner, it is indeed the forces of disease steering him. It is not uncommon for those patients who are most difficult to put up with, to suffer the most from their own disease.

4. It is not physical strength that counts in the nursing care of the mentally ill. The institutions need understanding, kind and experienced nursing staff. In most cases it is possible to calm agitated patients with skillful diversion and it is not necessary to resort to violence.

5. The nursing staff must be patient, friendly and accommodating to each patient equally and make allowances according to status and education. It is an easy task to behave with kindness and patience towards patients, who are receptive and grateful for such treatment. However, it is difficult to remain friendly and patient towards those patients who are agitated and disagreeable, and who reject with disdain any attempts to improve their situation ...[55]

---

[55]The excerpt is taken from the "Instructions" issued by Gudden to his nursing staff at the Upper Bavaria District Mental Asylum, in 1884. Hanns Hippius, Hans-Jürgen Möller and Gabriele Neundörfer-Kohl (eds.), *The University Department of Psychiatry in Munich: From Kraepelin and his Predecessors to Molecular Psychiatry*, chapter 4. Heidelberg, Springer (2008).

6 The Tragic Deaths of the King and the Professor

According to Wolfgang Gudden, a fourth-generation descendant of Bernhard Gudden, Bernhard's appointments in Munich were supported by, and possibly instigated by, Bavaria's royal family.[56] In any case, just weeks after Gudden's arrival, the king let it be known that he had a "great desire" for Gudden to "periodically visit his Royal Highness, Prince Otto." Otto (full name, Otto Wilhelm Luitpold Adalbert Waldemar von Wittelsbach) was Ludwig's brother, and sadly, Crown Prince Otto was not well. As Ludwig explained in his note to Gudden, Otto had "for a long time ... been suffering from nervousness as well as hallucinations." He probably had progressive paralysis of the insane – or simply, progressive paralysis – a rather common illness at the time. Gudden accepted Ludwig's request and began looking after Otto. According to Gudden's biographers,

> Right from the beginning Gudden and some of his co-workers regularly visited the ailing Prince Otto at the Palace of Nymphenburg and later at the little castle of Fürstenried. Gudden wrote to the Queen Mother, Marie of Bavaria and mother of King Ludwig the Second, about these visits and their correspondence continued for the following fourteen years.[57]

In reality, it was not Gudden, but Gudden's students, nicknamed the "prince's doctors", who were taking turns looking after Otto. Franz Nissl, a recent medical school graduate and one of Gudden's favorite students, was one of these men. Two years earlier, Gudden had awarded Nissl a prize for the best neuroanatomical research. Now, to encourage Nissl's scientific interest, Gudden set up a small laboratory at *Schloss Fürstenried* so that Nissl could pursue his research when off duty from his caretaking responsibilities. Gudden himself seldom went to Fürstenried, preferring instead to remain in Munich, close to the hospital and the university.

---

[56] A. Danek, W. Gudden, and H. Distel (1989), p. 1350.

[57] From H. Hippius et al. (2008), chapter 4, p. 23.

Gudden and his students continued looking after Otto for another fourteen years. Then, on a June morning in the year 1886, Professor Bernhard Gudden, head of psychiatry at Ludwig-Maximilians University and director of the Upper Bavaria District Mental Hospital, convened a small meeting in his office. The men had gathered at the request of the Ministry of State of Bavaria to evaluate the mental status of their king, Ludwig the Second. More precisely, they had been asked whether the king was fit to rule. Gudden was the logical choice to head the inquiry because it was he who had initially voiced concern about Ludwig's mental health at a meeting with ministerial officers two months previously. Moreover, Gudden was still caring for Ludwig's younger brother, Otto, at *Schloss Fürstenried*. So, whereas it was Ludwig who had first called upon Gudden to care for his brother, it was now Gudden who was to investigate the sanity of Ludwig himself.

The meeting regarding the fate of Ludwig was held at the university. Besides Gudden, three of Gudden's professional colleagues attended: Dr. Hubert von Grashey, professor at the University of Würzburg; Dr. Friedrich Wilhelm Hagen, professor at the University of Erlangen; and Dr. Max Hubrich, director of the district mental asylum at Werneck. Gudden was well acquainted with all three men. His own university appointment had come at the expense of Hubrich, the man whom the university had initially appointed in the mix-up mentioned above, and Grashey was Gudden's son-in-law.

Gudden took his place behind the desk, while the others gathered in front. Light from the rising sun penetrated weakly through the heavy curtain draping the single window, providing a dim backdrop to the somber occasion. The committee members lit their cigars and briefly exchanged pleasantries before turning to the business at hand. They had before them the king's medical history as well as statements from eyewitnesses regarding the king's behavior, the latter compiled by Count Max von Holnstein, the king's attendant. From these documents they learned that Ludwig hated administrative work and that he preferred chatting with laborers than negotiating with statesmen. Admired by the common man, he was regarded as a fool by the educated classes which, unfortunately, were the only classes that mattered. As for the king's personal habits, his servants reported that he dined outdoors in frigid, cold weather and wore heavy winter clothing in mid-summer. These witnesses also recounted his crude and juvenile table manners, his abusive treatment of servants and his extreme shyness in the presence of unfamiliar persons.

Most damaging of all was Ludwig's well known penchant for building extravagant castles, among which the magnificent Neuschwanstein castle perched on a rocky crag in the northern Alps. The castle was inspired by Ludwig's musical friend, Richard Wagner, and more specifically by Wagner's operas. In one of his letters to Wagner, Ludwig wrote, "It will remind you of *Tannhäuser* (Singers' Hall with a view of the castle in the background) and *Lohengrin* (castle courtyard, open corridor, path to the chapel)."[58] In addition to Neuschwanstein, there was a huge palace at Herrenchiemsee and a ridiculous winter garden atop his Munich palace. For the latter, Ludwig had instructed his workmen to provide a landscape complete with a small lake, a boat, a large panoramic painting of the Himalayan Mountains, an Indian fisherman's hut, a Moorish kiosk and an exotic tent. The committee also learned that Ludwig had sent an architectural advisor and three assistants to India for the sole purpose of examining the cornice of a palace under construction in a remote village.

Such extravagance clearly pointed to a man obsessed with daydreams and fantasies. Moreover, as Gudden's little committee knew all too well, these buildings did not come cheaply. In fact, the total cost was nearly fourteen million marks. It was understood that Ludwig's friends and allies were prepared to help pay off the debt, but it was equally well understood that any request for that aid would come at the expense of Bavaria's reputation.

It did not take long for the eminent psychiatrists to conclude that Ludwig was mad. Nor did they waste much time in discussing which specific mental illness he suffered from. Certainly Gudden felt neither the need nor the desire to come up with an actual diagnosis. Keeping strictly to the terms of the mandate, it was enough for the committee to declare the king unfit to rule. The official report, which the men unanimously agreed upon, was short and to the point.

1. His Majesty is in a very advanced state of mental disorder and most probably suffering from what psychiatrists refer to as paranoia (insanity);

2. With this type of illness, with its gradual, but advanced development and the fact that it has been noticed for quite some time, His Majesty is to be declared irrevocably ill, and it is possible that his mental condition will deteriorate;

3. Due to his illness, it is clear that His Majesty no longer has his own will and for this reason is most likely to be unable to

---

[58]Clara Tschudi, *Ludwig II of Bavaria.* Lulu.com (2015), p. 249.

govern, and that this situation will most likely last not only a year, but for the rest of his life.[59]

With Gudden's report in hand, state authorities commissioned Ludwig's friend, Count Max von Holnstein, to raise a small posse for the purpose of retaining Ludwig. They found him at his yet unfinished Neuschwanstein castle. Their first attempt to capture him was thwarted when a group of armed citizens confronted the commissioners at the castle gate. As more local people gathered intent on protecting the king, the commissioners hustled Ludwig into the gatehouse. Baroness Spera von Truchsess, a forty-seven year-old woman, attacked the commissioners with her umbrella. A new detachment of police arrived at four o'clock in the morning, and they dispersed the crowd. The commissioners bundled the king into a carriage and drove him some ninety kilometers north to Berg Castle, a large but otherwise unpretentious structure beside Lake Starnberg. There, Ludwig was incarcerated. With the crown now vacant, Ludwig's uncle, Prince Luitpold, was appointed Prince Regent, ruler of Bavaria.

It should be noted that no member of Gudden's committee had interviewed His Majesty, and three of the four psychiatrists had never spoken a word to him. Only Gudden had briefly encountered Ludwig, at a formal reception some twelve years earlier. Nor had any representative of the king been present to defend him. Nevertheless, on the word of the four committee members, King Ludwig was disposed of his throne and locked up. Such was the power of German psychiatrists in the late nineteenth century. Although the medical specialty of psychiatry was in its infancy, its practitioners were already wielding the power long enjoyed by other medical professionals.

Gudden was assigned to manage Ludwig's psychiatric needs, so he spent the night at the castle. With the stressful events of the preceding days now behind him, Gudden looked forward to a short period of relaxation. Lake Starnberg was – and still is – a beautiful place. With Munich within easy reach by horse carriage, Gudden planned on dividing his time between Berg, where he would look after Ludwig, and Munich, where he would attend to his responsibilities at the university and the hospital.

On the morning following Gudden and Ludwig's arrival at Berg castle, the two men agreed to take a walk along the banks of the lake. Did the doctor ask the patient, or was it the other way around? No one knows

---

[59]From the report, "Medical expertise on the mental condition of His Majesty the King, Ludwig the Second of Bavaria," June 8, 1886.

for sure. Regardless, Gudden summoned one of his assistants, Dr. Franz
Müller, and told him of the plan. Müller asked Gudden if he could join
them, but Gudden said no, explaining that their patient was unstable and
fearful, possibly even paranoid. Since Ludwig did not know Müller, Gudden
thought it prudent to leave Müller behind. He told Müller that he and
Ludwig would return within two hours. Dr. Müller wished the professor
and the disposed king a pleasant walk, then watched as they disappeared
behind a strand of spruce trees.

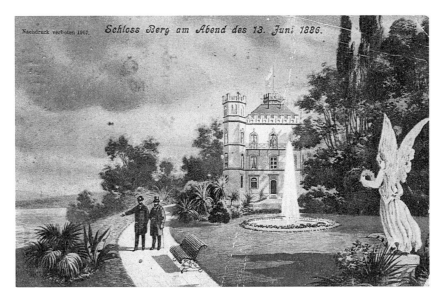

Figure 7: Contemporary postcard depicting King Ludwig II and Bernhard
Gudden on their fateful walk beside Berg Castle. [Wolfgang
Sauber (Xenophon)]

A full two hours later, Ludwig and Gudden had not yet returned. When
four more hours had passed with still no sign of them, a search party was
dispatched. In heavy rain and howling wind, the men carried torches along
the dark shores of Lake Starnberg. They searched in vain for several hours
until one of the men found something interesting.

Rushing into the waist-deep water, they found the motionless bodies of
Dr. Bernhard Gudden and King Ludwig II. Autopsies performed a few days
later showed that Gudden had suffered a blow to the head, and there were
marks around his throat suggesting strangulation. Ludwig had no marks
and, strangely, no water in his lungs. What happened?

The autopsy report led people to believe that Ludwig died of natural causes, perhaps from a heart attack. But that was obviously not the case with Gudden. Questions were raised. Was there a struggle? Did someone murder Gudden? Did they murder Ludwig? Did Gudden die while trying to stop his patient from committing suicide? In Munich, the cafes buzzed with rumors and conspiracy theories. Some people said that Ludwig was not actually dead but had fled to America with a large sum of money. A local fisherman, who claimed to have witnessed the events, left a note before his death describing the king's attempt to escape, followed by gunshots fired from the shore. According to this scenario, Gudden was killed because he was a witness to the king's murder. It is widely assumed that the autopsy was fraudulent and the authorities tried to cover up evidence. True or not, the cause of the tragedy at Lake Starnberg remains unknown to this day.

$$-//-$$

The ordinary citizens of Bavaria knew nothing of Gudden, but they mourned the loss of their king. The psychiatrists, on the other hand, were deeply affected by Gudden's sudden death. Not only was Gudden a respected leader, he was also well liked personally. His efficient hospital management and humane treatment of patients were widely admired and emulated. However, it was his mentorship of students that most affected the development of psychiatry. He influenced them by what he taught as well as by what he intentionally did *not* teach – as I will explain below.

Gudden worked at a time when the notion of mental illness as a brain disorder was being hotly debated. It was a scientific hypothesis that Gudden believed to be true, and he demonstrated his commitment to it by conducting his own neuroanatomical research. Although he was not alone in doing so, few professors of psychiatry trained as many students and assistants as did Gudden. Several of Gudden's research collaborators became prominent neuroanatomists in their own right. The flip side of Gudden's devotion to anatomical science was that he ignored certain clinical issues that weighed heavily on the minds of his fellow psychiatrists. Foremost among these issues was the problem of diagnosis. Hospital wards everywhere held a bewildering variety of psychiatric patients. It was no longer acceptable to simply call them "mad". In the medical climate of the late nineteenth century, it was considered desirable (but not always necessary) to attach a disease name to each patient's suffering. Practicing psychiatrists found this a daunting task because there were no good guides for distinguishing between different mental disorders, especially since the disorders were poorly defined. The problem of disease identification was also linked to another problem – how to represent all known mental illnesses in an orderly classification that reflected their fundamental similarities and differences. These two problems occupied the minds of many scholarly psychiatrists, but Gudden blinded his eyes and shut his mouth to both. It would be fair to assume that Kraepelin's own passion for clinical psychiatry grew, at least in part, from Gudden's unapologetic disinterest.

As I have explained, Gudden is important for reasons other than discovering new diseases or inventing better treatments. He did none of that. Nor did he get involved in contemporary discussions about diagnosis and classification He was a smart, capable man who could have done any of that, but he chose not to. Instead, he concentrated on anatomical research. His disregard for the intellectual challenges of clinical practice highlights the disconnect between clinical and biological approaches that prevailed in his day and that persists to a large extent today.

7 A Mismatched Pair of Rising Stars

Emil Kraepelin and Franz Nissl first met in Munich, probably in Gudden's neuroanatomy laboratory. Kraepelin was there examining reptilian brains, but he soon gave it up in favor of clinical work. Nissl, on the other hand, never left the lab. They tackled the mysteries of mental illness from different directions and had little in common at the personal level, yet they bonded strongly as colleagues and friends. Each found success in his own manner.

Nissl was born in Frankenthal on the banks of the Rhine River, in 1860. A quiet town in the Grand Duchy of Baden, Frankenthal was renowned for its elegant porcelain works – figurines, table wares, and the like. Baby Franz came into the world with a large, purple-pink mark on the left side of his face, and it never disappeared. It probably embarrassed him, and it was possibly the key to Nissl's awkward, sometimes brooding, personality. The mark might even have been a factor in the family's move to Freising, close to Munich, when Franz was just two years old. As an adult, Nissl habitually tilted his head in such a manner as to present the unblemished side toward interlocutors and photographers.

Franz's father, Theodor, worked as a middle school teacher. He was a religious man with intellectual pretentions. Franz's mother, Maria, had no such fancy interests. She was a soft-spoken woman devoted to her children. Theodor, however, was in full control, governing the family with a stern hand, even wielding the hand in a disciplinary manner at times. Because there was a chronic shortage of money, there was also friction and unhappiness, and that eventually brought Maria down with a case of "nervous illness". It was a nebulous diagnosis, often employed euphemistically to mask a case of suspected insanity. Maria was sent to the mental asylum at Illenau. Franz, then a young boy, visited her at the asylum on several occasions, accompanied by his aunt. It was his first contact with psychiatry, and likely formative. After several weeks of treatment with baths, Maria's condition improved, and she was released. However, when she later died, Franz was left with no protector. Theodore's new wife fared no better than Maria, and she took out her frustrations on the children, treating them coldly and singling out Franz's younger sister, Susanna, for physical abuse.

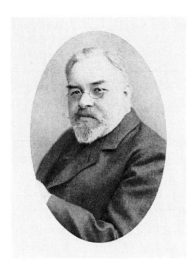 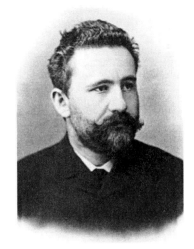

Figure 8: Franz Nissl. His facial blemish was evidently brushed-out by the photographer.

Figure 9: Emil Kraepelin, 1884.

Throughout these troubles, Theodor kept a close watch on Franz's schooling. He insisted that Franz read widely in both the classical and contemporary literatures. He hounded Franz about his unruly behavior and his disappointing school performances. Theodor was preparing Franz for priesthood, but Franz resisted, countering that he wanted to be a doctor and that he wanted to study in Berlin. An argument ensued, after which Theodor consented to medicine, but emphatically protested against Berlin, because Prussia was Protestant and the Nissls were Catholics. In the end, Franz enrolled as a medical student at Munich's Ludwig-Maximilians University.

Emil Kraepelin was four years older than Nissl. He came from a proudly Prussian, bourgeois family that celebrated every Prussian military victory and every expression of political influence. Kraepelin's father, Karl, was a music teacher, actor and occasional opera singer. Unlike Nissl's father, Karl left his youngest son to his own devises. After schooling in his hometown of Neustrelitz, Emil did his compulsory military service. He then studied medicine in Leipzig and Würzburg before taking his first professional job at Gudden's hospital. He was a robust-looking man with penetrating brown eyes, thick eyebrows and a furrowed brow. In manners, he was cool and reserved.

Growing up as a young boy, Kraepelin spent many happy days together with his brother Karl, who bore the same name as their father. Karl was ten years older than Emil and set on becoming a botanist. He already knew the names of all the plants and trees in the nearby woods, and he delighted in showing off his knowledge to his younger brother. At home, Karl fired Emil's imagination by telling him stories of wild animals in faraway places. He also performed tricks with chemicals, such as changing the color of crushed buckthorn berries from dark purple to red by adding lemon juice or, alternatively, changing the color to green by adding baking soda. Karl even tried to explain Charles Darwin's theory of evolution. In sum, Karl showed Emil how to view nature through the lens of science. Seeing the natural world as orderly and understandable was to become the guiding principle of Kraepelin's psychiatry.

Nissl was a southerner, a Bavarian Catholic. Kraepelin was a Protestant from northeastern Prussia. Nissl and Kraepelin were close colleagues, but they had very different personalities. Kraepelin was confident, strong-willed and decisive; Nissl was playful, self-doubting and lacking in polished manners. Kraepelin was also consistently well dressed, whereas Nissl was indifferent to fashion. Unlike in so many respects, one thing they had in common was the pain of estrangement from their fathers. In each case, it happened near the start of their medical studies. Kraepelin's father left his family to indulge in theatre and booze, while Nissl's father abandoned Franz on account of what he perceived as Franz's incorrigible liberality. Another thing they shared was the habit of hard work.

Kraepelin and Nissl met sometime in 1881. Kraepelin was an assistant physician at the Upper Bavaria District Mental Hospital, and Nissl was a medical student. In the following year, Kraepelin went to Leipzig, but he returned to Munich one year later. By that time, Nissl was in his final year of medical studies, but spending most of his time at *Schloss Fürstenried* looking after Otto, the king's insane brother.

Kraepelin became keenly aware of his younger acquaintance when it was announced that Nissl had won a prize for the best student thesis. It was a prize awarded by Gudden, who was now Dean of Medicine. Although Nissl was to continue his anatomical research for another thirty-five years, scientists know him today mostly for the work described in that student paper. It was research on the brain, but it stemmed directly from Robert Koch's research on bacteria. Why that was the case, requires explanation.

Koch was a physician who served as a surgeon in the Franco-Prussian war. After the war, while working in the German province of Posen (now part of Poland), he set up a research laboratory and taught himself how to grow colonies of bacteria. As a result, he was able to isolate the bacterium that causes tuberculosis. It was a breakthrough discovery, because tuberculosis was a major health concern at the time, responsible for one of every seven deaths in Germany. Koch announced his discovery at a meeting of the German Physiological Society in Berlin, on March 24, 1882. It was attended by thirty-six men, including the esteemed Rudolf Virchow, master of cell biology. Koch's lecture was published seventeen days later in the *Berliner Klinische Wochenschrift* (Berlin Clinical Weekly).

> I began my investigations, using material in which the infective organism would surely be expected, as for example in fresh growing grey tubercles from the lungs of animals which had died three to four weeks after infection ... Earlier observations having shown that in certain cases the deepest staining and clearest differentiation of bacteria from surrounding tissues were yielded by the use of the alkaline reaction, advantage was taken of this fact.[60]

Koch's description of his methods pointed to the "alkaline reaction" as the key to his success, and it would likewise become the key to Nissl's success. The chemical process to which Koch referred was a chance discovery, made three decades earlier by an English teenager named William Perkin. The boy had been encouraged by his teacher at the Royal College of Chemistry to experiment with coal tar to see if he could use it to make quinine. Perkins took up the challenge in his own laboratory located in the family home. Since quinine was needed for the treatment of malaria, there was money to be made from a cheap source. Making it from coal tar, however, was a dangerous business, because Perkin needed a substance called aniline, which had to be separated from benzene, a known explosive.

At one point, while working to obtain aniline, Perkin found that he had produced a black goo. Trying to purify it - or perhaps just trying to clean up - he added some "spirits of wine", which turned the substance a purplish color. Perkin dipped a piece of silk into the thick liquid and watched as the cloth turned brilliantly purple. Remarkably, the color did not wash out,

---

[60] Alex Sakula, "Robert Koch: Centenary of the discovery of the tubercle Bacillus, 1882," *Canadian Veterinary Journal* 24:127-131 (1983), p. 128.

nor did it fade in sunlight. In short, Perkin's experiments had yielded a synthetic dye that was attractive, easy to make and cheap. Moreover, it turned out that dyes of many different colors could be produced by making small changes in the chemical process. From that day forward, clothing manufacturers no longer had to rely on plant and animal dyes.

Robert Koch realized that aniline dyes might be useful for staining biological tissues, so he purchased a small quantity of methylene blue from Friedrich Bayer, the owner of a small chemical company that later sold billions of aspirin pills. The results were spectacular. Since the dyes are alkaline, they stick to acidic bacteria, and Koch's tubercular bacteria showed up blue. Shortly after Koch's discovery, his talented assistant, Paul Ehrlich, used a different aniline dye, magenta, and got even better results. Magenta gave the bacteria a bright purple-pink color. Ehrlich enhanced the effect by staining the non-bacterial tissue with aniline yellow and heating the slides.

Learning of Koch's and Ehrlich's successes in staining bacterial cells, Nissl realized that those same aniline dyes might work equally well with brain cells. He chose to experiment first with Ehrlich's magenta dye. In the beginning he used animal brains, but later, during an eight-month period of intensive work, he stained more than one hundred human brains. Results from initial trials were disappointing. The nerve cells were only faintly colored, and they faded with time. A legend tells of Nissl watching a colleague throw microscope slides into a sink full of soapy water before cleaning them. Somehow, Nissl got the idea of adding Venetian soap to his staining solution *et voila*! – those slides did not fade. The results were stunning and unprecedented. In contrast to other methods, which stained only slightly, Nissl's method left every nerve cell vividly colored. Moreover, Nissl's method revealed certain structures lying *inside* the cells that no anatomist had ever seen before.

Nissl immediately recognized the nucleus and, within it, the smaller, darkly stained nucleolus. Looking more closely, he noticed something unusual. Clustered around the nucleus, in every cell, were many tiny particles. At first, Nissl did not know what to make of them. He was skeptical, thinking they could be artifacts, but what he saw was real. Today, we know these particles as the rough endoplasmic reticulum, also called Nissl bodies or Nissl granules. These organelles contain large amounts of RNA, the substance that directs the making of proteins. Similarly, the nucleolus contains large amounts of DNA, which holds the body's genetic code. Since RNA and DNA are both acidic, and aniline dyes react strongly with acidic structures, Nissl's method worked especially well for highlighting the

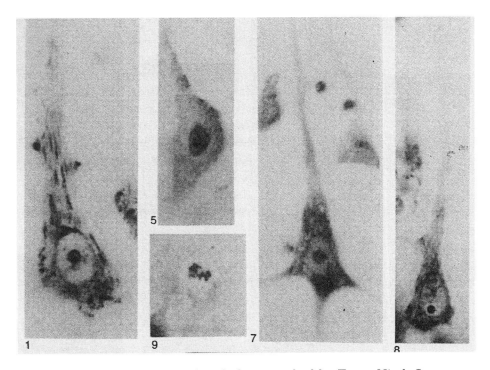

Figure 10: Nerve cells stained and photographed by Franz Nissl. Image no. 1 is a healthy cell, all others are from a patient with progressive paralysis of the insane. [Kraepelin's textbook, 1899]

endoplasmic reticulum and the nucleolus. Nissl knew nothing about RNA or DNA, but he did imagine that the small structures now visible in his microscope might hold clues to the cause of mental illness.

Kraepelin, along with everyone else, thought Nissl's slides were marvelous. He surely noticed, though, that the pink color of the stained nerve cells perfectly matched the color of the blemish on the left side of his friend's face.

Nissl, of course, was delighted with Gudden's prize. It was the ticket to his future career as a neuroanatomist. And yet, he could not quench his doubts. Did the cells really look like that in the living brain? Could he be certain that the much-talked about clusters of particles were not artifacts of the chemical technique? Also concerning were comments that he had overhead referring to poor writing in his report. Some people thought it unreadable. Others found fault with his methods. Whether he anticipated such a reaction, or whether he was simply expressing his own doubts, he proclaimed at the very beginning of the report, that "the stamp of incompleteness, of unfinishedness, is present on every page."

Nissl's thesis was titled, *Results and Experience in the Investigation of Pathological Changes in Nerve Cells of the Cerebral Cortex*. Regardless, most of the pathology described in the thesis related not to nerve cells, but to blood vessels and glia cells, the latter being a type of non-neuronal, supportive cell common in the brain. As well, nothing was clearly linked to mental illness, because Nissl provided no information about the patients whose brains he examined. While most of the specimens probably came from patients who had died with progressive paralysis, but there must have been brains from patients with other mental illness, and possibly some who had died of physical illnesses or old age.

Nissl became fixated on aniline dyes and used them almost exclusively for the remainder of his career. Sadly, though, he never found what he was looking for – abnormalities in the structure of nerve cells that could be definitely associated with mental illness. Modern neuroanatomists still use aniline dyes, or "Nissl stains" as they are called. They also have newer stains and sophisticated techniques for examining cellular inclusions. However, neither Nissl bodies nor any other intracellular structure has yet been found to correlate with any mental illness. The neuroanatomical correlates of psychiatric illness lie more in the structure of neuronal fibers, which were invisible with Nissl's stain.

Robert Koch and Paul Ehrlich won Nobel Prizes (at different times and for different works), but Franz Nissl won no more prizes after the one given to him by his mentor, Bernhard Gudden. Viewed in their totality, Nissl's anatomical accomplishments were not nearly as important as Emil Kraepelin's clinical insights, but Nissl's story is also the story of neuroscience in its early days, and neuroscience ultimately became as relevant to psychiatry as clinical observation.

–//–

While Nissl was settling into his career as an anatomically-minded psychiatrist, Kraepelin was headed down a different path. His was a broader, more intellectual vision of psychiatry. Keenly aware of the scientific revolution happening around him, he wanted to be part of it – not as a laboratory researcher, but as a clinician and an academic. Already at age twenty-two, he set himself the goal of becoming a professor by the age of thirty. As things turned out, he was two months late.

Kraepelin states in his *Memoirs* that he stopped studying reptile brains because he had a visual defect that prevented him from seeing clearly through a microscope. Whatever the reason, it was a wise decision, the proper one for a man with ambition. Kraepelin tackled some of the biggest issues then besetting psychiatry, and he brought them to ground, even if he did not forever quiet them.

He prepared for his life's work by reading the textbooks of Pinel, Esquirol and Heinroth. He bought into Griesinger's argument that mental illnesses must, somehow, be brain illnesses, but he doubted that neuroanatomy could provide all the answers. He reckoned that there was more to mental illness than brain pathology alone. Consequently, he thought a lot about the mind (*der Geist*); he thought much less about either the soul (*die Seele*) or the brain.

One can only imagine Kraepelin's excitement in the early days of his work at the Munich hospital. Walking through the wards accompanied by his supervisor Gudden, he would have encountered the full gamut of psychiatric illness. Many years later, Kraepelin recounted the experience,

> The confusing throng of demented, sometimes unapproachable, sometimes obtrusive patients, with their ridiculous or repellent, pitiable or dangerous oddities, the futility of the medical treatment, which was usually limited to salutations and the clumsiest bodily care, the complete helplessness against these types of insanity, for which there is no scientific explanation, made me feel the entire rigor of my chosen profession.[61]

These vivid impressions inspired a desire to learn more about individual patients, to gain insights into their bizarre behaviors, and to understand their differences. Although it may have seemed at times that every patient was unique, Kraepelin knew that there were names for some of the conditions – mania, melancholia, dementia and so on – even if he did not really understand what those terms meant. The descriptions, or diagnoses as some would call them, were imprecise and inconsistent from author to author. Were they fundamentally different disorders, even actual diseases, or were they just shorthand summaries of signs and symptoms? Kraepelin, the psychiatrist, retained the teachings of his brother regarding all the different plant and animal species dwelling in the forest. He realized that psychiatry had a long ways to go before joining botany and zoology as a

---

[61]E. Kraepelin (1987), p. 11.

scientific discipline. Whereas those other fields had long ago identified their types, psychiatry had yet to do so.

Not only did he fail to find guidance in the older textbooks, he was also disappointed to learn that Gudden had little interest in matters pertaining to diagnosis. Apart from administering the hospital and providing basic medical training, Gudden's attentions were focused on neuroanatomy. Maybe he found clinical issues too fuzzy. Maybe he preferred working with his hands over delving into arcane texts. Whatever was the case, his disregard for diagnosis, let alone classification, was obvious in the way that he taught his students. Kraepelin captured the essence of Gudden's attitude in this memory,

> The doctors from the wards were often quite surprised about the disclosures their patients made during the clinical instruction. However, after explaining the individual case, Gudden made no attempt to make any general clinical observations. He only really made one single diagnosis with certainty, namely that of paralysis [progressive paralysis of the insane], which he based on physical symptoms. He doubted and did not accept attempts to define other clinical syndromes or to trace the fine differences in the mental behavior; he avoided any questions in this context and repeated the answer, 'I do not know'. He preferred to leave such problems to the 'sublime beings'.[62]

Kraepelin must have found Gudden's attitude puzzling, but equally, as an ambitious man of science, he must have recognized the opportunity. If not Gudden, then why not himself to untangle the mess of psychiatric diagnosis? For that purpose, however, he needed to become a professor, for only as a professor could he hope to obtain resources sufficient for his purposes. Every university in Germany had but one professor of psychiatry, and he (always a man) automatically became director of the university's clinic. The twin positions provided a constant supply of patients, student researchers and professional assistants, all of whom Kraepelin would need to achieve his goals.

When Kraepelin finally did get his first professorship, at Dorpat (now the city of Tartu in Estonia), he was asked to give an inaugural speech. It was, for him, a special occasion and he took the opportunity to speak freely about the kind of psychiatry that he wanted to pursue as a doctor-scientist.

---

[62]E. Kraepelin (1987), pp. 13-14.

He began with an honest appraisal of psychiatry's current status. "If one surveys the various medical disciplines," he said, "it is surprising to find that nowhere are the directions of research so many and so varied as in psychiatry – a discipline which doubtless has the lowest academic standing."[63] In his opinion, the main difficulty lay in the "impossibility of a satisfactory solution to the fundamental psycho-physical problem." He said that mental illnesses are not brain diseases in the sense that physiological events *cause* mental events. Rather, in his view, physiological events and mental events occur independently, in parallel, with no causation in either direction.

He denounced "naïve materialism" and declared that a full understanding of psychological phenomena would never be achieved by investigations limited to anatomy, physiology and pathology. And, he bluntly stated that no significant advances in understanding mental illness had yet come from any of those approaches. "Although we are able to make at least some sense of the disease processes in the brains of paralytics, we most certainly lack hard facts about insanity, and no less about melancholy and mania." While agreeing that brain science might someday be useful to psychiatry, he stressed the need for a "proven relationship between a simple and unequivocal observation of anatomical pathology and an equally simple and unequivocal observation of psychological pathology."

In this last assertion, Kraepelin echoed the skepticism of Karl Kahlbaum, an asylum psychiatrist from an earlier generation. Kahlbaum was a solemn, pedantic man whose theoretical contributions were not fully appreciated until long after his death. Kraepelin, in particular, borrowed many ideas from him. Around the time that Gudden and Griesinger were beating their drums for brain anatomy, Kahlbaum wrote these cautionary words about the potential of neuropathology,

> This work has produced much valuable material but contributed nothing to the basic views on the origin of mental illness or on the anatomical locus of their diverse and significant manifestations; the view is now spreading that only comprehensive clinical observation of cases can bring order and clarity into the material ... It has now been recognized that it is futile to search for an anatomy of melancholy or mania, etc. because each of these forms occurs under the most varied relationships

---

[63]The quoted passages are taken, with minor editing, from the English translation of Kraepelin's lecture. Eric J. Engstrom, *History of Psychiatry* 16:350-364 (2005).

and combinations with other states, and they are just as little the expressions of an inner pathological process as the complex of symptoms called fever.[64]

Kraepelin concurred in Kahlbaum's tempered view of neuroscience. However, he was fudging his bets, because he would soon hire Franz Nissl to work on precisely the same problems that Kahlbaum had denounced.

After finishing his introductory remarks, Kraepelin spoke at length about his self-declared main interest, clinical diagnosis. He pointed out what must have been obvious to at least some in the audience, namely, that the categories of disease currently in use were inexact and confusing. Then, in a statement that straight went to the heart of his approach, he said, "Psychiatrists are unable to locate the essential and characteristic aspects of an individual case because they are lost in a labyrinth of clinical symptoms."

His use of the phrase, "essential and characteristic aspects", is significant and was no doubt intentional. Ever since Plato and Aristotle, western philosophy had entertained the proposition that every kind of thing has its essence, a set of properties that make that thing what it is. For example, one can say that the essence of silver lies in its molecular structure. Knowing this, we can predict the temperature at which silver melts, its hardness, et cetera. The same can be said for giraffes. Their essence is long legs, a long neck and patchy coat coloring. Any individual animal that one would wish to call a giraffe, must possess these essential features. Kraepelin believed that mental illnesses also had their essences, and that they lay deeper than superficial symptoms.

Next, Kraepelin again dismissed what he called the auxiliary disciplines of psychiatry, namely, chemistry, neuroanatomy and pathology. "None of them," he said, "is directed at what should be the common goal, namely the *clinical* study of mental disorders, or the empirical determination of individual forms of madness according to their cause, course and conclusion [italics in original]." He urged his fellow physicians to seek out and identify those "natural symptom clusters" which are the true pathological expressions of psychological processes. "Psychiatrists should not be allowed to duck the responsibility of describing mental processes and conditions in a manner consistent with the science of psychology."

By these statements, Kraepelin voiced his conviction that psychological insights, rather than anatomical or physiological data, would provide the

---

[64]Karl. K. Kahlbaum, *Catatonia.* Baltimore, Johns Hopkins University (1874, 1973), p. 2.

keys to clinical diagnosis. From that day forward, he put aside not only neuroanatomy, but also skull measurements, blood pressure measurements, biochemistry and other conventional medical tools. He did not completely neglect them, but they became of secondary importance. For, Kraepelin, the key to a deeper psychiatry lay in clinical observation and psychological research.

At the close of the Dorpat lecture, Kraepelin put all his comments into perspective and ended on an optimistic note,

> For the time being, it will be clinical observation in the strict sense of the word from which we can expect tangible progress in our scientific knowledge. But over the subsequent course of our development there will come a point in time when clinical observation alone will no longer satisfy our scientific aspirations. At that point, the ephemeral disputes between individual research directions will dissolve into mutual support and assistance, and all the divergent paths will again converge on one another in order to achieve one common goal: a natural science of mental illness.

8 Experimental Psychology

Kraepelin described himself as a "pure psychiatrist with psychological tendencies," which is apt in light of the projects that he undertook in the early years of his professional life. First, there was clinical work to discover the "essences" of mental diseases, and second, psychological research to expose the "inner pathological processes" characteristic of those diseases. These were ambitious projects even for a man of prodigious energy, and success was not assured.

Kraepelin used an interesting phrase in his Dorpat lecture, when he mentioned the "science of psychology". The word psychology, like psychiatry, comes from the Latin *Psyche*, which corresponds to mind. Psychology, then, is *the study* of mind. In speaking of the "science of psychology", Kraepelin was literally talking about "the science of the study of the mind." He no doubt felt it necessary to emphasize that psychology *is a science*. Speaking as he did in the year 1886, psychology had been scientific for less than ten years.

People must have studied minds – their own as well as other people's – ever since the origin of the human species, or at least since we got our minds. The reason we got them in the first place was for self-reflection and to aid us in navigating our social environments. Intellectuals have written about the mind for centuries. It was called philosophy. Psychology as a distinct field entered the picture only in the early nineteenth century, when commentators began using such terms as "lawful" and "scientific" in relation to mental events. Some authors put forth serious proposals about how experience shapes thoughts. But psychology was still being done while sitting in a soft chair, curved tobacco pipe in hand. It lacked two essential features of scientific activity: experiments and numbers. Emmanuel Kant, probably the most influential philosopher of the eighteenth century, had insisted that the mind could not possibly be studied with mathematics.

Pushing Kant aside, *physi*ologists (not *psych*ologists) around the middle of the nineteenth century started using quantitative methods in their investigations of vision, hearing and other senses. Psychologists were interested in that work, but they claimed a distinction between sensations and perceptions. Sensations are immediate and raw, they said, products of the physical brain. Therefore, sensations could be studied physiologically. Perceptions, on the other hand, are interpretive and come from the intangible mind. Since the mind functions in a manner totally unlike the brain, it is beyond the reach of any experimentalist.

A discovery by the physiologist, Hermann von Helmholtz, a former student of Johannes Müller, changed all of that. In 1849, Helmholtz startled everyone by announcing that he had measured the speed at which electrical signals (action potentials) travel in the nervous system. It was not absurdly fast, as many had believed, but rather, at the comfortable rate of about thirty meters per second (in the frog's sciatic nerve). Suddenly, it became imaginable that perception, and perhaps other psychological phenomena, might be measurable after all.

Next came Ernst Weber and Gustav Fechner, a teacher-student pair working at the University of Leipzig. They wondered if it would be possible to measure perceptions. They set up experiments in which, for example, several stones of known weights were successively placed in a subject's hand. Suppose the first stone weighed one pound. The subject might say that it felt light, and when pressed to give the perception a numerical value, she might say (arbitrarily), "two". Now, a weight of four pounds was placed in her hand. After comparing the second weight with the first – in her head – she described the second weight as two and one-half times heavier than the first, or five on the arbitrary scale. The surprising result came when she was presented with a sixteen pound stone and reported that this third stone again seemed two and one-half times heavier than the second stone. Thus, despite the fact that the third stone was *physically* sixteen times heavier than first stone (16 pounds versus 1 pound), the *subjective* weight had increased only six and a quarter times (12.5 versus 2.0).

From experiments like the foregoing, Weber and Fechner devised a psycho-physical law which says that the strength of a subjective sensation is proportional to the *logarithm* of the stimulus intensity, not the *linear* ratio, as one might naively assume. The Weber-Fechner law has been tested numerous times and it is remarkably accurate, not just for weights but also for sounds and lights. Suddenly, psychology had become quantitative. Moreover, it had been demonstrated that genuine experiments were as doable in psychology as in any other scientific discipline.

Although Weber and Fechner get credit for those milestone experiments, the man most responsible for establishing the "science of psychology" was Wilhelm Wundt, and it was to Wundt's laboratory that Emil Kraepelin went to learn about psychological experimentation. Going there was a bold decision. It would have been bold for any man at the beginning of his career, because the future of experimental psychology was uncertain, but for a psychiatrist, it was unprecedented.

Kraepelin had been working in Munich as assistant physician under Bernhard Gudden. In 1882, he left to be tutored by Wilhelm Wundt. It was a dream come true for Kraepelin, who had first learned of Wundt's work while in university. There, he had read a series of articles published under the title, "On the Souls of Humans and Animals". Later, after reading Wundt's *Principles of Physiological Psychology*, published in 1874, Kraepelin knew that he would eventually study with him.

Wundt was a professor at the University of Leipzig. Born into an academic family, he presumably learned from his parents the two keys to a successful academic career: write well and publish often. In both respects Wundt lived up to his parents' expectations. By the end of his long career he had written at least twenty-five books, many of which came out in multiple volumes and successive editions. He was a soft-spoken, kindly man possessed of enormous energy and creativity. In photographs, his long beard, wire-rimmed spectacles and soft eyes speak of a quiet dignity.

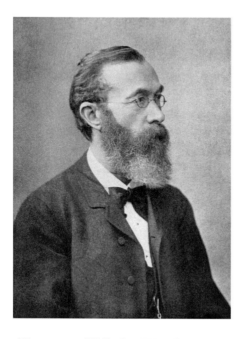

Figure 11: Wilhelm Wundt, 1902.

Wundt's *Principles of Physiological Psychology* is a large, impressive work that contains much description of nervous system structure and function. More interesting for the modern reader is the Introduction, in which Wundt spells out his overall agenda. Lacking neither hesitation nor modesty, he declares in the very first sentence, "The work which I here present to the public is an attempt to mark out a new domain of science."[65] He goes on to say that "psychology ... seeks to give an account of the interconnexion of processes which are evinced by our own consciousness."

Although interested in consciousness, Wundt rejected introspection, the investigative method favored by most of his fellow psychologists. Introspection, he said, leads to distorted conclusions because the observer and the observed are united in the same person. By contrast, "The great importance of the experimental method ... lies not simply in the fact that ... it enables us arbitrarily to vary the conditions of our observations, but also and essentially in the further fact that it makes observation itself possible."

Wundt also rejected the faculties of mind concept advanced by Aristotle and Kant. For him, "The uselessness of the faculty-concepts is almost universally conceded." Instead, he thought of the mind as a collection of "processes", where each process is responsible for performing a specific task. "There is, to be sure, no special faculty of ideation or feeling or volition; but the individual idea, the individual affective [emotional] process, and the individual voluntary act are looked upon as independent processes, connecting with one another and separating from one another as circumstances determine." The job of the experimental psychologist was to study the processes one by one, each in isolation from the others. Inspired by the physiologists, he chose to study the processes involved in sensation and perception.

Wundt established the Institute for Experimental Psychology at Leipzig University in 1879. Equipped with the very best instruments and headed by a charismatic leader, it quickly drew young men from around the world. There were philosophers, school teachers, managers and psychologists from many different backgrounds, but only one doctor, Kraepelin.

Kraepelin's decision to move to Leipzig was all the more impressive for the precarious circumstances of his career at that time. He was attracted almost equally to psychiatry and psychology. In which field should he specialize? His decision to leave Munich for Leipzig sprang from a notion

---

[65]Quotes here and below from Wilhelm Wundt, *Principles of Physiological Psychology*, 5th ed., translated by E. B. Titchener. London, Swan Sonnenschein (1902, 1910), pp. v, 1, 5, 19-20.

of what might be an ideal professional life. He would work as a psychiatrist to earn a comfortable income, but concurrently work as a professor at a university so that he could pursue his scientific work. For the plan to succeed, however, he would need the *Habilitation*, an advanced certification required of all high-level university appointees.

Candidates for the *Habilitation* had to submit a lengthy research-based dissertation, evidence of additional scholarly works and letters of recommendation. The final test was an oral presentation. Kraepelin wrote to Wundt asking him if he would supervise research that could form the basis of his *Habilitation*. Wundt wrote back saying that he would be happy to do so, but he could only provide a half-salary. Fortunately for Kraepelin, one of Wundt's colleagues, a doctor named Paul Flechsig, offered Kraepelin a part time job as his medical assistant. It looked like the perfect situation – allowing Kraepelin to pursue his psychiatric work *and* his scientific work – but it ended badly.

In the period of Kraepelin's stay at the Institute, Wundt was busy measuring sensory reaction times, meaning the minimum time required for a subject to press a button after seeing something or hearing something. Earlier, he had discovered that the delay for a simple reaction is longer than the time required for a nervous impulse to travel "up" from a sense organ to the brain and then "down" to a reacting muscle. He concluded from this fact that a large portion of the total reaction time must be due to processes occurring within the central nervous system – *mental* processes, as he understood them.

Meanwhile, a Dutchman, Franciscus Donders, had come up with a clever way of determining exactly how much time is consumed by a single mental process, specifically with respect to those processes active during reactions. In one such experiment, Donders had his subjects perform two types of reactions, one in which the subject was instructed to respond as quickly as possible after seeing or hearing a stimulus, and a second type in which the subject had to choose between different stimuli before responding. By subtracting the time for the simple reaction from the time for the more complex reaction, Donders was able to measure the time elapsed during the mental process of sensory discrimination. The method became known as "mental chronometry".

Wundt thought that the instrument Donders was using for recording reaction times was clumsy and maybe inaccurate, so he asked a master craftsman to build a better one. Soon he had an instrument that was accurate to one thousandth of a second; he called it the chronoscope. With

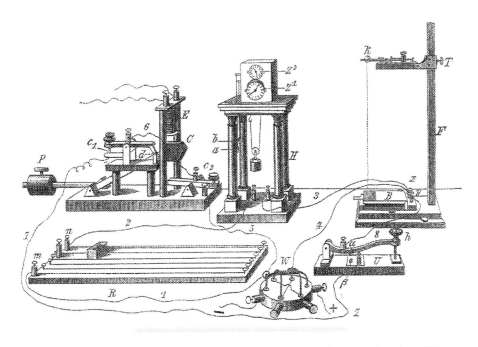

Figure 12: Wundt's reaction time apparatus. F, auditory stimulus; W, see-saw switch; C, Kontrollhammer; H, Hipp chronoscope; R, rheostat; U, response key. [W. Wundt, *Grundzüge der physiologischen Psychologie*, 5th ed., v. 3, 1902-03]

this excellent instrument in hand, and cognizant of Donders' successes, Wundt designed experiments to study various mental processes, including sensory recognition, acts of will and decision making.

In one such experiment, he determined the time required for completing tasks that varied in their complexity. For this, he had his subjects listen to recognizable sounds. In early trials, they listened to just one sound, later a few, and eventually many sounds. After the sound(s) stopped, Wundt asked the subjects to identify the sound(s) that they had heard. Not surprisingly, the more sounds the subject heard, the longer the time required to name them. He also studied word associations. After pronouncing a single word, he asked his subjects to signal the moment when he or she thought of a second word that was somehow associated with the first word. One student at the institute tested a large number of subjects, finding that the time required to make an association ranged between 707 thousandths of a second and 874 thousandths of a second.

While Wundt instructed Kraepelin in the goals and methods of experimental psychology, he also spoke to his student about the nature of mind and its relation to the brain. Most Europeans accepted Descartes' concept of the mind as a kind of "substance". They also followed Descartes in believed that the mind and the brain interact in a reciprocal, causative manner. Some intellectuals, however, held to other concepts of mind. Wundt believed in parallelism, a mind-body philosophy adopted, with modifications, from earlier German philosophers. In Wundt's philosophy, there is always a *correlation* between mental phenomena and physical (brain) phenomena, but not necessarily a *causation*, either from brain to mind or vice versa. Wundt did not discuss whether the mind is spiritual, substantive, or something else. His philosophy was intended only as an aid to the interpretation of his experimental results. Kraepelin bought into this point of view, but unlike Wundt, who did not hesitate to expound on "psychophysical parallelism", Kraepelin seldom wandered far from the laboratory or the clinic.

Wundt asked Kraepelin what kinds of experiments he would like to do. Given Kraepelin's dual interests in psychology and psychiatry, and knowing that he believed in psychological pathology, Wundt no doubt expected Kraepelin to conduct experiments comparing reaction times in patients and healthy subjects. As it turned out, Kraepelin did not do any experiments of that type until several years later, and the results were disappointing. He found that the reaction times of manic patients and aphasic (language impaired) patients were longer and more variable than those of healthy subjects. From those results, he drew the fuzzy conclusion that "the flight of ideas [characteristic of manic patients] was not the accelerated consequence of mental images, but of volatile and unstable emerging processes in the conscience."[66]

Rather than looking at patient reaction times, Kraepelin told Wundt that he wanted to study how drugs affect reaction times in healthy subjects. The idea was to simulate the mental processes of psychiatric illness. He spoke about the possibility of model psychoses, mental states similar to those of a psychiatric illness, but pharmacologically induced in healthy subjects. He would measure the drug effects under controlled conditions using Wundt's scientific methods. Wundt consented to Kraepelin's proposal. Aware of the novelty of his plan, which was indeed a new field of medical/scientific investigation, Kraepelin coined the term, pharmacopsychology. It is known today by the same term, but in reverse: psychopharmacology.

---

[66]E. Kraepelin (1987), p. 44.

Kraepelin chose to begin with alcohol. Later, after moving to Dorpat, he would test other drugs including tea, amyl nitrite, chloral hydrate, chloroform, ethyl ether and morphine. His subjects performed simple visual and auditory reactions, first before they had drunk any alcohol, and then again after drinking alcohol in different concentrations. The experimental design was simple, but the results were inconsistent. As the experiments proceeded, Kraepelin became concerned about possible problems. He realized, for example, that he might be biasing the results by testing the subjects with drinks that were *progressively* stronger, so he mixed up the order of the alcoholic solutions. He also added raspberry syrup to the solutions to improve their taste. And, curious as to whether the reaction times might be affected by the carbonic acid present in the drinks or by the feeling of a full-stomach, he performed a few experiments substituting carbonated water for alcohol. This last innovation may have marked the first use of a placebo control in pharmacological research. In total, he completed forty-seven experiments using four subjects, one of whom was himself. Summarizing these experiments, Kraepelin wrote that alcohol produced

> ... a slowing of intellectual processes with very fast onset and relatively slow remission ... a simultaneous facilitation of movement initiation appeared that lasted for a maximum of 20-30 min and was followed by an aggravation in the same domain. Higher doses caused an earlier onset and more extended occurrence of impairment, also in the motor domain. The [author] deduces from these experimental experiences the well-known picture of acute alcohol intoxication in all details and demonstrates how alterations in associative processes, the occurrence of stereotypes, sound associations, and insinuations of flight of ideas can be interpreted as motor excitements.[67]

Forsaking quantitative analysis almost entirely, Kraepelin based his conclusions mostly on his own experiences as one of the subjects. He was honest enough to acknowledge the extremely high variability of reaction times, writing,

> I was then not yet aware of the amount and irregularity of normal fluctuations in long-lasting psychometric experiments and

---

[67]U. Müller, P.C. Fletcher and H. Steinberg, "The origin of pharmacopsychology: Emil Kraepelin's experiments in Leipzig, Dorpat and Heidelberg (1882-1892)," *Psychopharmacology* 184:131-138 (2006), p. 133.

therefore did not take the necessary precaution. Consequently, we have to admit that some alterations of reaction times related to alcohol might be independent from the drug and caused by different influences.[68]

All things considered, it would be fair to conclude that nothing of lasting value came from these particular experiments.

After finishing with alcohol, Kraepelin prepared to move on to other drugs that might better mimic the effects of psychiatric illness, but one of his employers intervened before he could get started. Evidently Professor Flechsig, who was paying one-half of Kraepelin's salary, had a history with Professor Gudden. A few years earlier, Flechsig had visited Gudden's neuroanatomy laboratory in Munich. Following the visit, Gudden learned that Flechsig had published a paper using some of Gudden's microscope slides, but without obtaining Gudden's permission. They were slides showing the precise origins of the corticospinal tract, and it was Gudden's discovery, not Flechsig's. Gudden expressed his displeasure at the time, and now Flechsig acted as though he was taking out his bitterness over the incident by firing Gudden's student, Kraepelin. After telling Kraepelin that he would be away for a fortnight, he remarked that he was leaving the lab in someone else's hands because he found Kraepelin unreliable. Ouch! Besides holding a grudge against Gudden, Flechsig may also have resented Kraepelin spending so much time in Wundt's psychology laboratory, when he should have been working in Flechsig's medical clinic.

The situation might have proven disastrous for Kraepelin had he not been determined to get his *Habilitation*. He dipped into his savings, obtained a part-time job in a neurology clinic, and persuaded Wundt to offer a larger stipend. With his financial security restored, Kraepelin completed the dissertation based on his experimental research. As well, he put together a collection of scholarly essays that he had written on topics as diverse as criminal psychology, ethics, aesthetics and humor. All he needed now for the *Habilitation* was letters of recommendation. Fearing Flechsig, he instead asked Wilhelm Wundt and Bernhard Gudden to vouch for him, and they submitted sterling endorsements. In due course, the Minister of Culture announced that Kraepelin had been granted the *Habilitation*. Everyone – with the possible exception of Flechsig – was pleased to hear it.

Once again, Kraepelin confronted a difficult career choice. He had envisaged a dual career as professor of psychology *and* head of an asylum

---

[68]U. Müller, P.C. Fletcher and H. Steinberg (2006), p. 135.

or clinic, but he now realized the impracticality of that plan. So, again the question, psychology or psychiatry? He was enthralled with experimental psychology and happy in the university environment. But, the low salaries paid to young professors would hardly allow him to marry and start a family. Psychiatrists were handsomely paid by comparison, and the jobs were generally secure, but the drawback here was that jobs in psychiatry were hard to find. In the midst of this personal dilemma, Wundt opportunely stepped in to offer advice as scientific mentor and surrogate father. He told Kraepelin that experimental psychology had not yet taken hold in academia, and that jobs in that particular field were, in fact, quite scarce. Arguing that psychiatry offered better opportunities, Wundt urged Kraepelin to look for a suitable position in that field.

Thrust into professional limbo, Kraepelin returned to Munich and again worked as an assistant physician in Gudden's hospital. (It was then that he learned of Nissl's prize for anatomical research.) After one year in Munich, he went to the city of Leubus, in the province of Silesia, now part of Poland. There, he worked as senior physician at a small asylum. The clinical work was light enough for him to complete some psychological experiments, so he extended his work on word associations and studied reaction times at different times of day. Confident now with respect to his finances, he married his childhood sweetheart, Ina. The ceremony took place in the Prussian village of Stavenslust near his hometown of Neustrelitz. It was time for them to build their family. Before they could do so, however, he was offered a position in Dresden. The pay was less than in Leubus, and he was not allowed to do any scientific work, but the job came with the opportunity to direct a department of psychiatry in a general hospital. This stop, too, turned out to be short lived, for he and Ina soon moved on. Just as well, because within a month of arriving in Dresden, the couple's first child, a daughter, was strangled to death by a twisted umbilical cord.

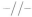

In the summer of 1886, the Kraepelins were vacationing in Switzerland when they heard the news of Wilhelm Gudden's death at Lake Starnberg. A few days later, they took a train to the German seaport of Stettin, followed by a steamboat to Reval (now Tallinn in Estonia), and then another train to Dorpat, where Emil had found a job as professor at the local university and, simultaneously, head of a mental hospital. At the train station in Dorpat, the Kraepelins hired a carriage to take them to the hospital. It was a short trip that nonetheless taught them much about the situation that they had gotten themselves into, because they found themselves unable to communicate with the carriage driver. Since they were both ignorant of the Estonian language, they had to ask a bystander to translate their instructions from German into Estonian.

The Hospital for the Mentally and Nervously Ill — Kraepelin called it the clinic — was constructed of wood. It comprised two floors and had a stone cellar. As in Germany, the structural plan was symmetrical: one-half of the building was reserved for women, the other half for men. Within each wing, one ward was reserved for "quiet" patients, a second ward for "agitated" patients, and a third ward for "raving mad" patients. Designed for fifty-six patients, there were about one hundred patients resident in the clinic when Kraepelin arrived. The high fees were usually paid for by the patients' families.

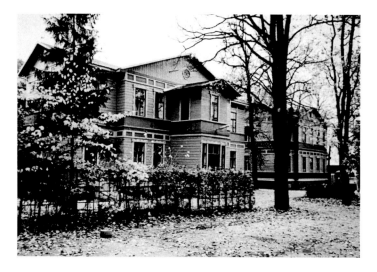

Figure 13: The psychiatric clinic at Dorpat, c. 1887.

Emil and Ina resided in a house adjacent to the clinic. The balcony of their new home afforded a view of a thick spruce forest and beyond that, across the Embach River, a cathedral tower standing tall above the town. Dorpat was a strange, multilingual town.[69] For centuries, it had been fought over and governed by several foreign peoples, including Swedes, Poles, Danes, Russians and Germans. It was now part of the Russian Em-

---

[69]For a full account of the linguistic situation in Dorpat, see M. Rotzoll and F. Grüner, "Emil Kraepelin and German psychiatry in multicultural Dorpat/Tartu," *Trames* 20(70/65): 351-367 (2016).

pire, but the German nationals, who made up less than six percent of the Estonian population, were effectively the ruling class. Times were changing, however, as the Russians pushed for greater control and, simultaneously, the Estonians sought to express their nationality. There was a struggle for language primacy. The majority of Dorpat residents spoke only Estonian. A few of Kraepelin's patients spoke Russian, Latvian or German, but Kraepelin spoke only German, so he was forced to use a translator in most cases. The translators were themselves Germans – Kraepelin's assistant physicians – whose knowledge of other languages was fragmentary. Hence, the vital business of interviewing patients took a great deal of Kraepelin's precious time, and it frustrated him no end.

Given the circumstances, Kraepelin felt more comfortable at the university, where all but six of the forty-six professors were Germans. The medical school was the largest, and by some accounts the most prestigious, in the entire Russian Empire. After delivering his inaugural lecture, the one in which he outlined his vision of a scientific psychiatry based on psychology and clinical observation, he settled into his work.

He made friends with Alexander Schmidt, a professor of physiology who also served as president of the university. Suspecting that Schmidt had little time for research, Kraepelin asked him if he would give up one of the rooms allotted to him so that Kraepelin and his students could use it for their experiments. Schmidt consented, Kraepelin ordered new apparatus, and soon the experiments were up and running. Kraepelin was overjoyed to finally have his very own research program. Excitedly, he wrote to Wundt,

> [The study] on the effects of exercise and tiredness has progressed the most. Here I had several processes which occur in daily life (reading, writing, counting, arithmetic skills, et cetera) systematically investigated. The aim was to obtain normal figures, to be used as the basis for investigations on sick people, for whom the more precise methods of time measurement [reaction times] were too difficult. It seems that coefficients for adaptation, exercise and tiredness can be calculated for every field and every individual, in which his recent state of mind as well as his energy in general will be reflected.[70]

---

[70]Quoted in Holger Steinberg and Matthias Angermeyer, "Emil Kraepelin's years at Dorpat as professor of psychiatry in nineteenth-century Russia," *History of Psychiatry* xii: 297-327 (2001), p. 306.

Kraepelin was now exploring new research grounds. Sensing that there was more to experimental psychology than reaction times and discrimination experiments, he looked for psychological processes that might be more relevant to psychiatry. With this goal in mind, he decided to study *work*, or more specifically, psychological work. How, exactly, work relates to mental illness is unclear, but apparently Kraepelin saw a connection. He devised a simple task for his experimental subjects that required them to execute a succession of simple arithmetic calculations, usually additions, within a preset time limit. Upon completion of the task, Kraepelin quantified the efficiency of the work by counting the number of calculations performed. Kraepelin expected that completion rates would vary between subjects, depend on the time of day, change during the course of testing, and be affected by personal factors. It was a pared down task suited to scientific analysis and capable, he thought, of revealing hidden psychological processes.

Kraepelin was anxious to share initial results with his fellow scientists. He wanted feedback (hopefully positive) and he wanted to promote the field of experimental psychology to a community that knew very little, if anything, about it. After all, it was an exciting, new field of science. By attracting other researchers to the field, he would not only help it grow, he would establish himself as one of its leaders. With these purposes in mind, Kraepelin founded the Dorpat Psychological Society.

In the beginning, the Society was quite small, consisting of perhaps a dozen men drawn from the German-speaking academic and medical communities. The first meeting was likely held in a café. There, the gathered men would have ordered beers and lit their cigars while waiting for their president to speak. After welcoming the members and making a few remarks on behalf of the Society, Kraepelin would have talked about his recent research.[71]

He probably started by explaining why he decided to study mental work, and why he decided to examine a very simple form of it. He would then have described the task that his subjects were asked to perform and, to make things easier for the audience, he may have shown them an example of the worksheets given to the subjects. It would have looked something like this, except much longer:

---

[71]My description of Kraepelin's work curves is based on his article, "Die Arbeitscurve," *Philosophische Studien* 19:459-507 (1902). Many of the experiments described therein were conducted in Dorpat, but others were conducted earlier in Leipzig, or later, in Heidelberg.

A	B	C
6	4	
2	7	
6	3	
7	8	
8	6	
4	2	
9	1	

His subjects started at the top of the sheet, adding the numbers 6 and 4 in columns A and B, and entering the sum 10 into column C. They were told to proceed down the sheet row by row, adding and entering the sums on each line as quickly as they could. Most sessions lasted one hour, but some went longer. At the end of each session, Kraepelin constructed an *Arbeitscurve*, or work curve. For this, he calculated the total number of items completed in successive five minute segments throughout the session. The work curve was a measure of the subject's mental performance over time. For members of the Dorpat Psychological Society, he might have passed around a second paper showing one or more work curves. Each curve formed a different pattern, but in every case the lines jumped up and down as they moved from left to right.

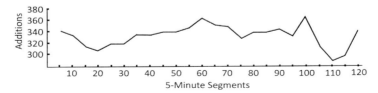

Figure 14: A typical work curve, reconstructed from examples illustrated in Kraepelin's monograph (1902).

Kraepelin was interested in the temporal fluctuations of performance during a single test session, that is, the up and down movements of individual work curves. He assumed that the shape of the curve was determined by interactions between multiple mental processes, and he analyzed the data in the hope of identifying the responsible processes. Most obvious were the effects of *practice* and *fatigue*. Naturally, practice improved performance (increasing the number of completed additions), whereas fatigue had a negative effect (reducing the number of additions). Kraepelin realized that practice and fatigue would act simultaneously, but with different time courses. Performances typically improved at the beginning of a session, due to practice, but then declined toward the end of the session when fatigue set in.

With further study, he found other influences on performance and, as with practice and fatigue, he assumed that each influence had its own time course. Initially, the subjects were uncomfortable, finding themselves in a novel situation. Hence, they began their work hesitatingly, and rates of performance were low. *Adaptation* to the task allowed their performances to gradually improve. *Incentive* also helped in the early stages, but it quickly faded, causing a downward movement in the curves. The fifth and final factor was *motivation*, which had a positive influence like incentive, but was longer lasting.

Looking at any single *Arbeitscurve*, such as the one shown in Figure 14, it is difficult, if not impossible, to detect the play of Kraepelin's five factors. Even if he were correct in claiming that these five factors – and only these factors – accounted for the shape of the curves, the simultaneity of their actions obscured their individual contributions. Kraepelin needed a method to separate the factors and delineate their unique time courses. He decided to introduce pauses during the tests, reasoning that a brief pause would relieve fatigue, but not greatly change the practice effect, and that other factors could be differentiated in a similar manner. He thought that by introducing pauses of various durations, he could isolate and characterize all five factors.

When presenting his work to the Dorpat Psychological Society, Kraepelin might well have held up yet another sheet of paper, showed it briefly, and allowed it to be passed around the audience. It would have been a table summarizing the results in from a single pause experiment (Figure 15).

Segment Number	1	2	3	4	5	6
Practice	0	56	96	133	167	199
Fatigue	0	41	82	123	164	205
Motivation	0	35	40	45	45	45
Adaptation	0	30	35	40	45	50
Incentive	90	0	-4	-15	0	-8

Figure 15: Results from the first thirty minutes of a pause experiment, reconstructed from Kraepelin's monograph (1902).

The thirty minute session was divided into five-minute segments. The numbers in each row show the strength of influence for each named factor in each five-minute segment. The trends are consistent with expectations. Practice and fatigue both have large effects that gradually accumulate, whereas motivation and adaptation have lesser, more steady influences. Incentive has the most dramatic effect, with a strong initial influence followed by a rapidly declining influence. Kraepelin would have emphasized his conclusion that the performance score for any given subject in any given five-minute segment depended on the particular combination of influences operating during that time. But questions would have been asked.

What, exactly, do the numbers in the table represent? How did he calculate them? How well does the analysis account for the shape of the *Arbeitscurve*? Why did he not use differential equations, a mathematical tool that was available at the time and that is ideally suited to sorting out the time courses of the individual factors? And, crucially, what is the relevance of any of this for psychiatry? Addressing this last question in his *Memoirs*, Kraepelin wrote only that, "They shed light on the traumatic neuroses and certain psychopathic conditions."[72]

Apparently oblivious to the flaws in his methodology, Kraepelin expanded his studies of work curves to include such mental tasks as reading, number learning and syllable learning. He continued these experiments until at least 1902, at which time he published a 50-page review of the work, which was dedicated to his mentor, Wilhelm Wundt (note 72).

The truth of the matter is that the *Arbeitscurve* added nothing to our understanding of either mental illness or psychology generally. It was an innovative research strategy, but fundamentally flawed in its conception and ineptly practiced. Max Weber, an influential social scientist and one-time patient of Kraepelin, roundly criticized the *Arbeitscurve* for its irrelevance and technical shortcomings. Among other comments, he noted the absence of incentives (especially economic incentives), and the fact that the laboratory environment in which the experiments were conducted was unlike real-life school and work environments.

The inconsequential results of Kraepelin's psychological experiments – encompassing reaction times, association tests, psychopharmacology and *Arbeitscurven* – does not detract from their historical significance. They marked Kraepelin's passage from traditional psychiatry to modern psychiatry, from the anecdotal consideration of individual cases to the scientific study of underlying causes.

---

[72]E. Kraepelin (1987), p. 45.

9 Kraepelin and Nissl in Heidelberg

Kraepelin kept busy in Dorpat with work curves, scholarly writing and hospital duties. Nevertheless, he was unhappy. First of all, he hated the long winters, which were much harsher than in Germany. The freezing temperatures and frequent snowfalls darkened his days. Besides that, there were the work-related frustrations. He struggled with money concerns, infrastructure issues, and the complications of caring for more patients than the small clinic could comfortably accommodate. Adding to his discontent was his wife's homesickness and their shared sadness over baby Marie's death in Dresden. Even after Ina delivered a healthy daughter, Antonie, in Dorpat, Emil's mood scarcely lifted. Hoping to refresh himself, Emil left Ina with the baby and took off on a long trip, visiting friends and colleagues in Austria, Switzerland, Italy and Germany. One highlight of the trip – noted in his *Memoirs* – was when he spotted a colorful frog near Vienna, picked it up and brought it back as a present for his brother Karl.

Upon returning to Dorpat, Kraepelin found that little had changed. He tried to get the government to help solve problems at the clinic, but communications between him and the bureaucrats were difficult, owing to the language barrier and thick layers of red tape. The Ministry of Education regularly balked at Kraepelin's urgent requests for additional funding, yet demanded report after report. Bad feelings went both ways. On one occasion, when the Ministry insisted that he submit certain documents in Cyrillic script (which he did not know), he flatly refused. That action so incensed the governor of Livonia that he sent Kraepelin an official order demanding that he obey the law.

Kraepelin was further crippled by cultural and linguistic incompatibilities. They interfered with his management of the clinic and, more significantly, they frustrated his attempts to interview patients. By imposing a distance between himself and his patients, they stymied his efforts to engage in the kind of psychiatry that he had promised in his inaugural lecture. He was anxious to tackle the problem of diagnosis, but he could not.

Ina gave birth to a third daughter, Vera. However, with the memory of Marie's death still fresh in their memories, tragedy struck again when Vera died on the last day of February, 1890. She was not yet two years old. And then, just twenty days after Vera's death, further disturbing news came from Germany. Otto von Bismarck, Kraepelin's lifelong hero, had been forced to resign his posts as Chancellor of Germany and Minister President of Prussia. Evidently the new Emperor, Wilhelm II, did not like Bismarck's politics. Numb from the cold and generally fed up with everything in Dorpat, the Kraepelins decided to go back to Germany. Unfortunately, Emil had no job to return to.

Kraepelin yearned for a well-funded, easily-governed clinic where he could pursue his scientific and medical interests. Of all the psychiatric institutions in Germany, only those affiliated with universities in the largest and most progressive cities fit the bill. If he were lucky enough to get an appointment at one of these universities, he would have the freedom and power to achieve his goals. Apart from the fact that he knew of no current openings, there was also the matter of qualifications. Would the German authorities look with favor upon his modest successes in Dorpat under trying conditions, or would they dismiss his work there as irrelevant?

One thing that Kraepelin had going for him was his publication record. Regardless of where he was living and what duties he had to perform, he always seemed to find time for writing. Adding to his output from Leipzig, when he was bulking up his credentials for the *Habituation*, he had since written articles on hypnotism, migraine headaches, false memories and pharmacopsychology, among other things. Some publications featured his own research results, whereas others provided timely reviews of controversial subjects. He even published a pamphlet on research methods for experimental psychologists.

Moreover, he had recently completed the manuscript for a third edition of his textbook. The original version was written while working in Leipzig at Wundt's Institute. A publisher approached him asking if he would be willing to write a small book on psychiatry. At the time, Kraepelin's post-school experience in clinical psychiatry amounted to just four years at the Munich hospital, plus his part-time work with Flechsig in Leipzig. Nevertheless, because he was short of money, he agreed to write the book. The *Compendium der Psychiatrie* (Compendium of Psychiatry) was a concise statement of current knowledge, rather than a guide to clinical practice. Nevertheless, it sold well, and Kraepelin was encouraged to publish an updated edition, which he did four years later, in Dorpat. This second edition was given a new title, *Psychiatrie: Ein kurzes Lehrbuch für Studierende und Ärzte* (*Psychiatry: A Short Textbook for Students and Physicians*).

Two years after that, while still in Dorpat, the third edition appeared under the same title, except that the word *kurzes* (short) had been deleted. In the end, there would be eight editions of the popular textbook published during Kraepelin's lifetime, plus a posthumous ninth edition.

Surely, he thought, no academic critic could complain about his scholarly production. Moreover, he figured that his recent trip to central Europe would help, since he had intentionally visited several influential German psychiatrists. Those contacts finally bore fruit just as the Kraepelins were facing the prospect of yet another winter in Dorpat. On the ninth of November, 1890, good fortune came not once, but twice. First, Ina delivered Hans, the couple's first son. And second, Emil received a telegram from Wilhelm Nokk, Minister of Education for the state of Baden, in which he informed Kraepelin that he would be the new professor of psychiatry at the University of Heidelberg. Nokk wrote that he wanted to free Kraepelin from the claws of the Russian bear.

The Kraepelins did spend a final winter in Dorpat. But the following spring, when their the train came to a stop at the Heidelberg station, they could not have been happier. Looking upwards, their eyes would have been immediately drawn to the crumbling walls of the ancient *Schloss* (castle), which stood watchful above the city. On the opposite side of the Neckar River lay the gentle, green slopes of Heiligenberg Hill. Situated in a magnificent natural setting and benefitting from a mild climate, Heidelberg was a thriving town of thirty thousand residents. It owed its wealth in part to tourism (on account of the castle), but mostly to its fine university. Although small in comparison with the University of Berlin, the University of Heidelberg was a proud institution with a history dating back to 1386. Its medical school was considered by many to be the best in Germany, and the psychiatric clinic, to which Kraepelin had come, had earned its fair share of that high reputation.

The town spread out along the southern bank of the Neckar River. Its *Haupstraße* (high street), was a grand passage that led from the town center directly to its main attractions, the *Schloss*, the *Heiliggeistkirche* (Church of the Holy Spirit), the *Marktplatz* (marketplace) and the *Rathaus* (town hall). Along this street, a constant stream of smartly dressed men and women paraded and shopped.

Eastward from the town center, continuing on the line established by *Hauptstraße*, ran *Bergheimer Straße* (mountain home street), where the Kraepelin family found its new home. The house was the official residence of the clinic director, and it was but a short walk from there to the psychiatric clinic. Kraepelin's clinic, together with the adjacent neurology clinic and the women's clinic, formed part of the university's medical campus. The rest of the university lay further east amidst the greater bustle of *Hauptstraße*. With the Neckar River flowing serenely just across the road at the rear of the clinic, and little commerce nearby, it was the ideal ambiance in which to mix academic science and clinical medicine.

Persons employed by the psychiatric clinic helped the family settle in. Unfortunately, while Emil and Ina were still unpacking a few days later, their son Hans died. Suffering from an illness that he had brought with him from Dorpat, he died at the age of exactly six months. The tragic event marred an otherwise joyous occasion, and it was especially grievous coming as it did only slightly more than one year after Vera's death. Altogether, Ina had by this time given birth to four babies, of which only four-year old Antonie was still alive.

One of Kraepelin's first tasks, and maybe his most important, was to hire his assistant physicians. Unfortunately, the psychiatrist who had been an assistant to Kraepelin's predecessor, committed suicide; it was said that he was afraid of becoming mentally ill. Kraepelin's first choice was a young psychiatrist named Gustav Aschaffenburg. Originally from Cologne, Aschaffenburg was very well educated, having studied at universities in Heidelberg, Würzburg, Freiburg, Berlin and Strasbourg. His father was an astute business man and Talmudic scholar. Aschaffenburg had a wide academic knowledge, but he also enjoyed working on the wards. His specialties were psychiatric diagnosis and classification, the very subjects that interested Kraepelin. Moreover, Kraepelin suspected that Aschaffenburg's dissertation on delirium tremens might prove useful for his nascent campaign against alcoholism.

Next, Kraepelin thought of Franz Nissl, his friend from Munich. Since it was mandatory for any clinic with high aspirations to have an active neuroanatomy laboratory, Nissl, an enthusiastic researcher, was the obvious choice. While clinical work was a secondary concern for Nissl, he was known to have a kindly manner in dealing with patients, so he could certainly help out in that regard. And finally, Nissl was a jolly fellow. It could not have escaped Kraepelin's attention that having Nissl near him could help balance his sometimes excessive seriousness. Kraepelin thought that Nissl would jump at the chance of leaving Frankfurt, where he now worked, for Heidelberg, which was close to Nissl's birthplace in the Grand Duchy of Baden. But, as Kraepelin was soon to learn, the situation was complicated.

Nissl moved to Frankfurt shortly after graduating from medical school. The job suited him well because his responsibilities were about equally divided between neuroanatomical research and patient care. Unmarried, he lived with his younger sister and his aunt. Since the sister managed the household and some of Franz's personal needs, Franz was free to work as much as he pleased. He made enough money in Frankfurt to support himself, his sister and his aunt. He even gave monies to his step-mother and step-siblings.

Moreover, Nissl had found in Frankfurt a psychiatrist whose passion for neuroanatomy was as great as his own. Alois Alzheimer had been working at the asylum as an assistant psychiatrist since the previous year. He, like Nissl, was a Bavarian and a bachelor. They got along exceedingly well, so much so that when Alzheimer married, he asked Nissl to be his best man at the wedding. The son of a notary, Alzheimer was large and tall and had a personality to match. Bowed over a microscope with his pince-nez hanging loosely from his neck and his ever-present cigar waiting patiently on the table top, he was the very picture of a nineteenth century anatomist. Being a good-natured fellow, he quickly learned to reciprocate Nissl's wry sense of humor. After marrying, he became a devoted family man, but that did not prevent him from spending plenty of time in the laboratory. It was the essential glue that bound him and Nissl. Working together, they investigated brain pathologies relevant to neurological and psychiatric disorders, principally progressive paralysis.

Considering all that he had going for him in Frankfurt, Nissl was naturally reluctant to leave. On the other hand, he knew the beauty of Heidelberg and he had great respect for Kraepelin. For these reasons, and others, he agonized about accepting Kraepelin's offer. Kraepelin wrote several letters to Nissl spelling out his offer, but only after several weeks had passed did Nissl reply.

In a single remarkable letter spilling out over sixty handwritten pages, Nissl rambled on about his circumstances and explained in repetitious detail the reasons for his hesitation.[73] Why should I, he wrote, exchange my safe position in Frankfurt for an uncertain one in Heidelberg? He laments the fact that he is thirty-five years old. Maybe it would be too risky to take a job that may not result in a professorship. If it were only a matter of effort, of energy, he might succeed, but other factors could intercede. His

---

[73]Nissl's letter is dated August 15, 1895. It is reproduced in full in W. Burgmair, E.J. Engstrom, and M.M. Weber (eds.), *Kraepelin in Heidelberg*. München, Belleville (2005), pp. 195-217.

boss suggested that his own ambitions might suffer from competing with Aschaffenburg. And what would happen in the event that he did not get a professorship? His dear sister, who so depends on him, would be left vulnerable. He would have to return to an asylum and probably remain there forever as a second class doctor. Or worse, he might have to work as a prison doctor.

If he did choose to go to Heidelberg, he continued, it would be so that he could continue working as a scientist. Even though he came into the world without much money, he would not accept Kraepelin's offer just for the money, or even for the prestige of a professorship. It would be because he was convinced that nerve cell research held the key to understanding mental illness. In one long aside, he expounded on the idea that each neuron has a function that is linked to its structure. He also expressed concerns over technical problems, and expounded on his persistent worry that living neurons might not have the same structures as dead neurons.

Near the end of the long letter, Nissl proposed to Kraepelin that they cooperate in creating a photographic atlas of the entire human cerebral cortex. It would show every individual nerve cell, whether healthy or in a pathological state. Researchers would be able to determine which regions of the brain are most susceptible to mental illness, and possibly discover specific types of cell anomalies associated with specific types of mental disorder, for example idiocy, psychosis, catatonia, et cetera. "Naturally," he wrote, "I would undertake this project only as a side-job [underlying as in the original]!"

On the whole, Nissl's letter was more a plea for sympathy than a strategy designed to improve the offer. Nissl had a complex mind that Kraepelin did not fully understand. He waited patiently while Nissl continued to negotiate, deliberate and fret. In the end, Nissl did go to Heidelberg, and he never looked back. Gustav Aschaffenburg came too, and any fears that Nissl and Kraepelin might have harbored over a possible rivalry between Aschaffenburg and Nissl quickly dissolved. His boss must have invented the rivalry as a device to retain Nissl in Frankfurt because, in reality, there was no basis for competition. Whereas Aschaffenburg liked working directly with patients and was fascinated by clinical issues, Nissl truly liked (loved?) only laboratory research.

Kraepelin arrived in Heidelberg after confidently transiting from Würzburg, where he attended medical school, to Munich, then Leipzig, back again to Munich, then Leubus, Dresden and lastly, Dorpat. Nissl, by contrast had remained in Frankfurt since graduating from medical school.

Kraepelin moved whenever he was presented with a better opportunity, whereas Nissl always acted with caution, carefully weighing his scientific ambitions against his personal security. Fortunately, when the balance of Nissl's interests tipped in favor of science, a special partnership was formed between him and Kraepelin. The period from 1886 – when Nissl came to Heidelberg – and 1903, when Kraepelin left Heidelberg for Munich, was especially productive for both men.

With only two floors of occupied space, the Heidelberg clinic was smaller and less imposing than the Munich hospital, but otherwise similar. It had several gardens behind the main building in which patients and staff could enjoy fresh air. Kraepelin reorganized the floor space by combining a few small rooms into two large "surveillance" wards, one for males and one for females. With these special wards, doctors could observe small groups of patients under controlled conditions. Each day, the clinic director and his assistants chose the patients that would be put in the surveillance wards. The selected patients received highly attentive care. In return, albeit unknowingly, they provided Kraepelin with the observational material that he needed for assessing the diagnostic categories of mental illness.

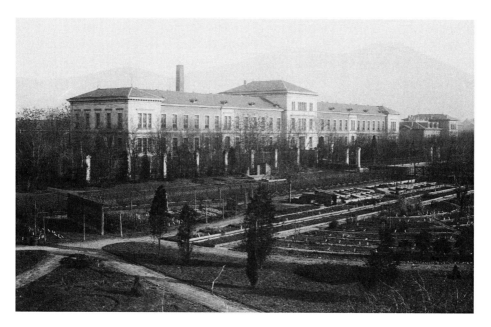

Figure 16: The psychiatric clinic at Heidelberg, about 1900. [Heidelberg University Library, Graph. Slg. A_0775]

Kraepelin quickly developed a fondness for Heidelberg, especially on account of its natural endowments. One of his greatest pleasures was walking on the sun-bathed southern slopes of Heiligenberg mountain. According to legend, it was a path that had been used by ancient poets and philosophers, who were inspired by its beauty. It was especially glorious in the spring, with the trees and flowers blooming, and the hairy stems of Pellitory-of-the-wall poking out from the brickwork along its borders. Just on the other side of the wall, lay productive vineyards, some dating from the seventeenth century. Walking accompanied by his Great Dane, Ramses, Kraepelin would stop at certain vantage points from which he could see the psychiatric clinic across the river.

Kraepelin came to Heidelberg with his goals intact but largely unattained. It was time to buckle down and tackle the related problems of how mental illnesses should be defined and they could be diagnosed. He was not ready to completely abandon the *Arbeitscurve*, but he started spending more time on the wards than in the psychology laboratory. With much relief, he was once again able to converse with patients in his native tongue. Still convinced that mental illnesses are "real things", like plants and animals, he set himself the task of sorting out what was true and what was false in the extant classifications.

According to his estimation, Pinel, Esquirol, Heinroth and all previous classifiers had met with only limited success. Collectively, they had named a plethora of disorders, but the usefulness of those names was compromised by the vagueness of the definitions and the lack of agreement among psychiatrists. Kraepelin saw a common method behind all earlier classifications, and it was faulty. Certain symptoms, such as hallucinations and delusions, were both obvious and common. Earlier authors, therefore, had either distinguished different forms of the dominant symptom – for example, intellectual mania versus emotional mania – or assumed connections between certain symptoms, naming them "symptom complexes" and likening them to illnesses.

Kraepelin rejected these classifications because they were based almost entirely on symptoms and unfounded speculations. Causes, courses and outcomes were for the most part ignored. Physical signs and biological markers were likewise rarely mentioned. Moreover, Kraepelin knew that some of the authors had only limited hands-on experience, whether in asylums or other institutions. Heinroth, for example, had little direct contact with patients, and Pinel, although he may have had in-depth familiarity with a few patients, probably had only patchy knowledge of the rest. Only Esquirol seems to have had substantial personal experience with the full gamut of cases.

Although Kraepelin's experimental work prior to coming to Heidelberg had been inconclusive, it gave him an acquaintance with scientific methods. He knew the value of data obtained by objective means. And, he realized that he needed more data from more patients. Anecdotal information of the kind collected by earlier psychiatrists would not suffice; he needed hard facts documented by trained observers. Nor was it enough to briefly interview a patient upon admission and then observe him or her only haphazardly afterwards. It was for this reason that he built surveillance rooms.

He also understood the need to sample the full range of psychiatric disorders, not just the most common types, or those manifested by individuals from a particular region, or of a particular social class. Unfortunately, most of the beds in the clinic were occupied by patients who had been there for a long time and who were destined to remain there, in some cases for the rest of their lives. Kraepelin knew that he could do little to relieve their suffering, and equally, that there was little more to be learned from them. He was frustrated by the fact that their dominant presence meant fewer opportunities for studying the less common disorders. Also, while he and his staff had ample access to late stage illnesses, they did not see enough of the early stages. For both of these problems, the obvious solution was to increase turnover by moving patients in and out of the clinic as quickly as possible. It was tricky, because it had to be done without overcrowding the clinic or jeopardizing the wellbeing of the patients.

Kraepelin set himself the goal of doubling the rate of admissions. Rather than simply taking patients when ordered to do so by state authorities, he began accepting voluntary admissions. He also arranged for transfers from jails when he learned of prisoners who might be especially interesting. No sooner had Kraepelin started implementing these changes, however, when he encountered resistance from government administrators. The clinic was governed by two authorities: the Ministry of the Interior, which was responsible for health care, and the Ministry of Education, which was responsible for medical training. His troubles with both ministries grew with time and eventually caused him to leave Heidelberg. The situation resembled Dorpat, and in both places the turmoil was fueled by Kraepelin's ambitions.

Friction between Kraepelin and the Ministry of Education first arose in connection with the transfer of patients from the Heidelberg clinic to the asylum at Emmendingen, a facility designed for the long-term care of chronically ill patients. Each transfer required a pile of paper work and then a long delay while bureaucrats reviewed the files. What really infuriated Kraepelin was the Ministry's insistence that they, not he, keep the patients' files. It was a matter of considerable importance because there was only a single copy of the files, and Kraepelin wanted to retain it so that he could track whether the patient improved or deteriorated. It was partly in response to this battle over government files that Kraepelin came up with his own plan for case documentation, one which proved to be very useful – perhaps indispensable – for his research into disease entities.

During his medical training, Kraepelin had worked at a psychiatric clinic in Würzburg, where one of his responsibilities had been to fill out a kind of census card for the government. The forms were called *Zählkarten*, or counting cards. They recorded the number of resident patients, their home locations, symptoms, duration of stay, curability, and if deceased, the cause of death. Collected from every asylum in Bavaria, the cards enabled the government to determine the geographical distribution of its patients and calculate statistics pertinent to planning and financing.

In Heidelberg, Kraepelin modified the cards to serve as research tools. He saw them as a means of documenting, and eventually categorizing, all the pertinent details of every patient's condition. In particular, he wanted them to contain information relevant to the diagnosis and subsequent course of the patient's disorder. Earlier psychiatrists, going back to Pinel and Esquirol, kept notes on selected patients, but Kraepelin's innovation was to standardize the procedure and collect key data on *all* patients, so far as possible. By going beyond the superficially "interesting" cases, he avoided biasing the observations. Also, to ensure scientific integrity, Kraepelin instructed his assistants and his students to focus on data of an *objective* nature, that is, to avoid *subjective* interpretations. Like an ornithologist intent on identifying and classifying all the birds present in a particular region, Kraepelin intended to use the *Zählkarten* for identifying and classifying psychiatric illnesses. In practice, however, it proved impossible to exclude all subjective judgments. One filled-out card from the Heidelberg clinic is shown Figure 17.

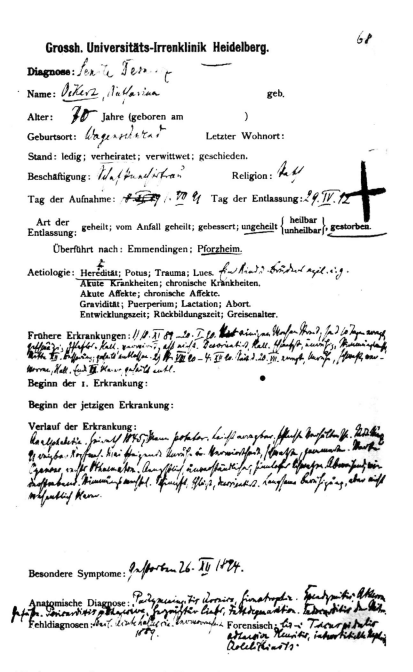

Figure 17: A page from one of Kraepelin's *Zählkarten*. [Archive Max-Planck Institute of Psychiatry MPIP-K20/SK VI]

Although most of the doctor's handwritten entries are illegible, the printed queries are clear. They translate as follows, from top to bottom:

Diagnosis

Name

Age

Birthplace/Last place of residence

Marital status (here, married)

Occupation/Religion

Date of admission/date of discharge

Type of discharge (here, incurable)/Transfer to (here, Pforzheim)

Cause of illness (here, heredity)

Early symptoms

First illness

Current illness

Course of the illness

Peculiar symptoms

Anatomical diagnosis

False (alternative) diagnosis/Forensic diagnosis

During the period 1887-1904, Kraepelin collected thousands of cards, corresponding to an equal number of patients. Whenever possible, he continued recording information even after the patient had been transferred elsewhere. For this purpose, he sent his assistants to neighboring asylums where they either interviewed the patient or simply read the updated file. Historians debate the extent to which Kraepelin actually relied on the cards for his definitions and classifications of mental illness. Later in this book, I will discuss the evidence.

$-//-$

Franz Nissl did not share his friend's fascination with the *Zählkarten*. His particular challenge was nothing less than understanding the human brain. He occasionally interviewed patients and thus filled out his share of cards, but given the choice, he preferred looking at microscope slides. Since his residence, laboratory and photographic studio were all located in the clinic's main building, he had little need to go elsewhere and he seldom did.

Nissl came to Heidelberg with no wife and no family. By choosing to live in an apartment located just above the neuroanatomy laboratory, he avoided any problems arising from working late nights in the laboratory. The apartment's large anteroom held Nissl's single treasure, a fine piano, which he played well. The bedroom doubled as a study. Someone had placed a crucifix on the wall above the bed, but Nissl was not very religious, so he removed the crucifix and replaced it with a framed text of his own composition. The text read, *ÉCRASEZ*, and underneath, *ROTTET SIE AUS*. The top line was taken from Voltaire, the eighteenth century French author. It referred to the command, *écrasez l'infame*, meaning "crush the infamous", an expression used by Voltaire when speaking of clergymen and royalty. The German expression *rottet sie aus* translates as "exterminate them", thus underscoring the sentiment expressed by Voltaire.[74]

Nissl's laboratory was a small, narrow room. It was furnished with three tables near the windows for students, and a separate work station for Nissl. Sharing space with the microscopes on the long tables were various tools and a scattering of glass slides. Chemicals, some powdered and some in solution, were neatly arranged in wooden cabinets. The range of color in the solutions (black, orange, yellow, red) produced a rainbow effect that brightened the otherwise drab decor. Larger jars stood on the open shelving. They held various body organs, both animal and human, some whole, some in pieces, but mostly brains. The air in the lab smelled strongly of acetic acid, carbolic acid, alcohol, kerosene, turpentine and other harsh substances. Throughout the day, and often at night too, the laboratory was a busy place, crowded with visiting scientists from England, France, Poland, Italy, Norway and America.

Because Nissl had promised Kraepelin a photographic atlas of the cerebral cortex, he set up a second research space in the clinic's basement that was specifically for photography. Kraepelin had been encouraging Nissl's use of photography ever since he saw pictures of nerve cells shown to him by a professor of zoology. No camera at the time could match the clarity, let alone the immediacy, of a brain slice viewed directly through a microscope, but brain slices were prone to drying out, becoming damaged, or fading so badly that it was difficult to see anything clearly. By contrast, photographs provided permanent records. The images were black-and-white and fuzzy,

---

[74]The description of Nissl's room, along with other personal details, is contained in C.B. Farrar, "I remember Nissl," American Journal of Psychiatry 110:621-624 (1954).

but what wonders they revealed! Furthermore, photographs could be sent to an interested colleague or even published in a scientific journal with worldwide readership, thus accelerating the dissemination of knowledge and, equally important, advancing the reputation of the anatomist.

Nissl's photographic lab was nothing more than a simple chamber of pasteboard walls placed inside a larger room. With the door of the chamber closed tight and the single lamp extinguished, the chamber was totally dark. The larger room outside the photographic chamber was occupied by a pharmacy and assorted medical devices.

In the center of the room was a long table upon which lay Nissl's microscope, a camera and associated optical devices. At the far end of the table stood a gas-fed lantern. Light from the lantern was shaped and focused by three condenser lenses positioned between the source and the microscope, the latter turned on its side. The light passed through the brain section, through the magnifying lens, and then through an eye piece lens at the far end of the microscope before entering the camera, which consisted of yet another lens, an expandable bellows and a glass plate coated with light-sensitive emulsion.

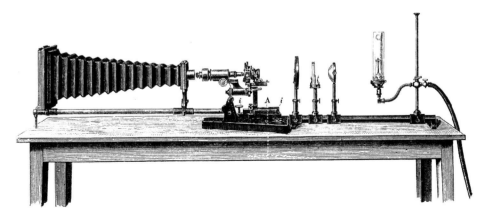

Figure 18: Photographic apparatus of the type used by Nissl. [Richard Neuhauss, *Lehrbuch der Mikrophotographie*, 2nd ed., 1898]

To take a photograph, Nissl worked alone in the basement, usually at night, fiddling with the often cranky apparatus. He first cleaned all the lenses with a chamois dampened with alcohol. Next, he ignited the light source by sparking a mixture of oxygen and hydrogen. The gases had to be mixed just right and turned on slowly, because there was a real danger of explosion. Once lit, the hot gas flame was directed to the base of a calcium oxide cylinder, which glowed with a pure white light, a limelight. Nissl shaped the limelight by adjusting the positions of the condenser lenses. Once he saw that the brain section was illuminated brightly and uniformly, he precisely position it and focused it. When satisfied with the preparations, he released the shutter. Depending on the thickness of the tissue section, the intensity of the light and other factors, the shutter would be kept open for as long as several minutes. It occasionally happened that men came to deliver coal during a photographic exposure. Since the furnace was situated near the photography lab, the coal, tumbling into its bin, rattled the timbers and shook Nissl's apparatus, thereby ruining his picture.

When one of his photographic exposures was interrupted by a delivery of coal, or something else went wrong in the laboratory, Nissl would shout out, *"Die Röhre ist gemotzt!"*. It was a verbal concoction with no literal meaning. Nissl liked playing with words, and the quoted expression contained two of his favorites, *die Röhre* and *die Motzung*. Both had multiple meanings depending on the context. *Die Röhre* translates as "the tube", and probably refers to a prominent part of Nissl's microscope. (His students called the cigars that he smoked, *Nissl-Röhren*). G*emotzt* is a corruption of the verb *motzen*, to complain. So, roughly translated, *Die Röhre ist gemotzt* meant, "The tube is garbage."

An American visitor to the lab reported another application of Nissl's linguistic creativity.[75] Once, when snacking at a café with colleagues, Nissl pointed to the salt container and asked his neighbor, *"Die Röhre, bitte* [Please pass the tube]. " After receiving the salt, and with no further pointing, he said, *"Jetzt, die Motzung,"* meaning "Now pass the pepper." Nissl's friends and colleagues became so accustomed to hearing *die Röhre* and *die Motzung* that they understood the intended meanings. Strangers, meanwhile, were befuddled.

The plan to produce a photographic atlas of the human cerebral cortex ultimately failed, not for lack of effort, but for technical reasons. The problem was, each photograph had to clearly depict every individual nerve cell while also encompassing the entire lateral extent of one-half of the brain. This would have required special lenses, finely grained emulsions and very large print sizes, none of which were available at the time. Although Nissl and Kraepelin were both disappointed, neither suffered from a lack of alternative projects. Moreover, one can speculate that the very idea of the atlas was only a ploy employed by Nissl during his negotiations with Kraepelin over the Heidelberg appointment.

---

[75]C. B. Farrar (1954), p. 623.

10 A Very Complex Thing

It has been claimed that the human brain is the most complex thing in the universe. The point could be argued, but certainly the brain is a *very* complex organ. You would hardly guess as much, looking at a brain collected at death. For starters, the actual brain would be buried beneath three layers of connective tissue and thus, invisible. Only if you carefully removed the connective tissue, would you see the creamy white brain. In this state, its most obvious feature would be the deep grooves, or fissures, that weave around its surface and define its lobes: frontal, temporal, occipital, et cetera. Its color and texture might bring tofu to mind, either soft tofu or hard tofu depending on how long the brain had been soaking in seventy percent alcohol. Although heavy in the hand, the brain's appearance would provide not the slightest hint of its complexity.

Réne Descartes was one of the smartest and best-informed intellectuals of the seventeenth century. In mid-life, he pondered the brain. He believed, from intuition, that the mind and the brain are different and separate. He thought, however, that they interact in the pineal gland. There, somehow, the mind governs the brain. For his description of how the brain works, he followed the example of the English physician, William Harvey, who had earlier described how the heart circulates blood. Descartes disagreed with Harvey's conclusions, but he was impressed with Harvey's focus on mechanisms. Thus, his take on the brain took the form of a hydro-mechanical model. Whereas Harvey got it right in explaining how the heart works, Descartes was woefully mistaken in explaining how the brain works.

> We see clocks, artificial fountains, mills, and similar machines which, though made entirely by man, lack not the power to move of themselves, in various ways ... Similarly, you may have observed in the grottoes and fountains in the gardens of our kings that the force that makes water leap from its source is able of itself to move diverse machines and even to make them play instruments or pronounce certain words according to the various arrangements of the tubes through which the water is conducted ... And truly one can well compare the nerves of the

machine that I am describing to the tubes of the mechanisms of
these fountains, its muscles and tendons to divers other engines
and springs which serve to move these machines.[76]

Descartes, like his contemporary Nicholas Malebranche and nearly everyone else at the time, believed that nerves were filled with animal spirits. A century and a half later, Luigi Galvani was dissecting a frog in Bologna, Italy. According to legend, he touched the exposed sciatic nerve with a metal scalpel that had inadvertently acquired an electrical charge – perhaps when Galvani brushed it across his woolen jacket. Immediately after touching the nerve with the charged scalpel, he noticed a jerking movement in the frog's leg. Galvani had discovered that it is electricity, not animal spirits, that animates nerves. After Emil Du Bois-Reymond discovered electrical pulses (action potentials), and his friend, Hermann von Helmholtz, measured the speed of their conduction in nerves, the problem of how nervous signals are transmitted over long distances was basically solved. Notwithstanding these advances, neuroscientists had not even begun to answer the really big questions.

The question that psychiatrists asked of the scientists was, What is wrong with my patient's brain? They expected to hear of lesions and structural abnormalities, but none were found. In the face of this fact, the more astute scientists realized that they had better look for more subtle aberrations. That endeavor required them to learn how the brain actually works, not necessarily in psychiatric patients, but in everyone. They reasoned that once they knew what the brain was supposed to be doing, they could go on to consider what it was *not* doing in the brains of patients. It was the correct approach, and it is the same approach taken today.

Neuroscience researchers at the time knew that the brain contains countless numbers of nerve cells and large masses of nerve fibers, but they had no real answers for how it controls even the simplest behaviors. The relationship between brain activity and normal mental activity was as much a matter of speculation in the nineteenth century as it had been for centuries past. Whereas neuroscientists today pursue such problems armed with genetic, molecular and whole-brain imaging tools, scientists in Nissl's day had relatively simple tools. A handful of scientists was experimenting with electrophysiological methods, but the majority stuck to their microscopes. What they lacked in instrumentation, they made up for in imagination.

---

[76]Réne Descartes, *L'Homme*, 1664 (posthumous).

Karl Wernicke – whose comments on the role of brain research I quoted earlier – was a psychiatrist, neuroanatomist and neurologist (a combination not uncommon in the day). A Prussian, he studied medicine at the University of Breslau (now the city of Wrocław in Poland), then worked in Vienna and Berlin before returning to Breslau as a professor. Extrapolating from earlier research, he came up with an idea that offered a framework for understanding how the brain works. Simply put, he proposed that each of the brain's functions is governed from a different region. It became known as the theory of cerebral localization. The idea was roughly similar to the phrenologists' concept of functional localization, but much more sophisticated because it was based on valid anatomy and realistic mental terminology. Wernicke was particularly interested in perception, intelligence and memory, each of which is affected by mental illness. Going further, Wernicke thought it would be possible to link specific psychiatric conditions (he called them symptom complexes) with specific areas of the brain. The proposal, and Wernicke's attempt to prove it, became the subject of much controversy.

Wernicke based his theory on the fact that the brain has parts. Viewed from the outside, the cortex, or cerebrum, lies above almost everything else. It is divided into left and right hemispheres. Each hemisphere is further partitioned into several large lobes including the distinctive frontal and temporal lobes. Other obvious structures include the cerebellum and the brainstem. Inside the brain, the hippocampus and the amygdala are distinctive.

Early in the nineteenth century, the Frenchman Jean Pierre Flourens sought to discover the functions of these parts. Experimenting on pigeons and rabbits, he systematically removed one or another structure and found that some did, indeed, have distinctive functions. When the cerebrum was removed, for example, the animals became blind, deaf and immobile. Contrastingly, when the cerebellum was removed, they lost their equilibrium and their movements became uncoordinated. If the brainstem was removed, the animals died.

Eduard Hitzig conducted further tests of localized function, particularly on the cerebral cortex. At the time, he was working as a physician with the Prussian army, and he was responsible for treating the wounds of soldiers who had been shot in the head. The bullets fractured the men's skulls, leaving Hitzig with the opportunity to experiment. He applied a weak electrical current at the points of fracture and discovered that stimulation elicited movements of the eyes and certain muscles. Upon returning to his laboratory in Berlin, Hitzig replicated and extended these results using dogs and applying currents directly to the brain. He was surprised to find that stimulation produced movements only when applied to a narrow strip of the cerebral cortex located at the posterior edge of the frontal lobe, an area now known as the "motor strip". He noted that the muscle movements occurred on the opposite side of the body to where the stimulus was delivered, implying a crossing of the motor fibers.

Hitzig became a psychiatrist only late in his career. He had been trained in internal medicine and knew little about psychiatry until he worked briefly at two asylums. Nevertheless, he was appointed head of a large hospital in Halle that had been built for the sole purpose of psychiatric research and education. Thus, Hitzig began as an internist, transformed himself into an electrophysiologist, and ended up as a powerful (but despised) psychiatrist. His career path encapsulates the late nineteenth century shift from asylum psychiatry to academic psychiatry.

Hitzig's experiments were repeated and extended a few years later by David Ferrier, a Scottish neurologist. Working with monkeys, he used weaker electrical currents than Hitzig, and he applied them with greater precision. These technical refinements led Ferrier to notice that movements occurred in different parts of the body depending on where, exactly, the motor strip was stimulated. For example, when the upper part of the motor strip was stimulated, the buttocks twitched; a little further down, the shoulder contracted. Towards the bottom of the motor strip lay the command centers for the elbow, wrist and fingers. This, at last, was convincing proof of localization, at least for motor control.

More information relevant to localization came from autopsies. Psychiatrists looked to autopsies not just to test broad theories of localization, but also for evidence of pathology, that is, damage or abnormalities in the brain that could explain their patients' symptoms. Already in the late 1850s, the deputy chief of psychiatry at the Charité in Berlin, Karl Westphal, was urging his younger colleagues to spend as much time at the autopsy table and the microscope as in the interview room. He cautioned them not to become discouraged if at first they found nothing of interest. Surely, if they looked more carefully, they would find evidence of localization.

> If during [the patient's] life we have observed a series of symptoms which can only be attributed to a disease of the brain and if upon death we find no macroscopic [large] sign of damage, then we shall always consider it desirable, that the entire

brain slice by slice, be subject to systematic microscopic investigation. This is because in spite of the integrity of its mass the most severe symptoms can potentially be the result of very circumscribed [minute] alterations.[77]

As more and more anatomist-psychiatrists began searching for neuropathy, the demand for brains increased. Soon, there were not enough brains for all the researchers who wanted them. After all, the supply was limited. Individual clinics started reserving beds for terminally ill patients and prohibiting their transfers elsewhere, for fear that they might lose the opportunity to perform an autopsy. Making matters worse, experimental physiologists also wanted cadavers, and they needed "fresh material". According to one report, a professor of ophthalmology informed an audience of psychiatrists and neurologists that he had found a way to elicit contractions of the eye pupil by applying electrical stimuli to the spinal cord. The report stated that the experiments were conducted on "two persons put to death by decapitation twenty-five and twenty-seven seconds respectively after the sentence had been carried out."[78]

A celebrated turning point in localization work came when the French neurologist Paul Broca examined the brains of two stroke victims who had lost the ability to speak. Remarkably, in each case he found damage limited to the bottom part of the left frontal lobe. Not long afterwards, Karl Wernicke, the outspoken champion of localization, confirmed Broca's findings in some of his own patients. He also found something quite different and very interesting. When he examined the brains of patients whose *speech* had been normal before death, but whose abilities to *understand* spoken words was severely impaired, he saw damage not in the frontal lobe, but in the upper portion of the left temporal lobe. Wernicke was naturally struck by the consistent relationship between the nature of the language deficit and the site of the lesion. These observations of Wernicke and Broca have since been replicated many times. It is a fact that language functions are mostly controlled from the left side of the brain, with speech *production* located in the frontal lobe and speech *comprehension* located in the temporal lobe.

Starting from these findings on language function, Wernicke proceeded to build a broad theory of cerebral localization that posited, among other things, specific locations for specific mental illnesses. However, some neu-

---

[77]Quoted in E. J. Engstrom (2003), p. 100.
[78]Quoted in E. J. Engstrom (2003), p. 103.

rologists pointed out that, even with respect to language dysfunctions, some deficits could not be explained by damage to either Broca's area (in the frontal lobe) or Wernicke's area (in the temporal lobe). A particular controversy arose over a rare condition involving patients who speak and comprehend normally but have difficulty in repeating phrases spoken to them by another person. Wernicke called the syndrome "conduction aphasia", and said that it was caused by a disconnect between Broca's area and Wernicke's area.

A young Viennese doctor by the name of Sigmund Freud took issue with Wernicke's interpretations. In 1891, he published a short monograph titled "On Aphasia: A Critical Study". Despite the fact that Freud was then *Privatdozent* (equivalent to associate professor) in the Department of Neuropathology at the University of Vienna, there is no evidence of him having examined any aphasic patient or even a brain taken from an aphasic patient after death. The book is based entirely on the published works of other authors. Although Freud was not completely opposed to the notion of localized functions, he rejected the Broca-Wernicke scheme for language dysfunctions, arguing instead for a more integrated model. In specific regard to conduction aphasia, he expressed doubt about Wernicke's claim that speech repetition could be lost while speech and auditory comprehension remained unaffected and, in any case, he refused to believe that it could be caused by the disruption of a fiber pathway, as proposed by Wernicke.

Wernicke did not give in to Freud's criticism. On the contrary, he seemed to feed upon it, spinning out even more detailed notions of localization. He wrote about a "sensory projection field", a "motor projection field" and a center of ideas. Further, he speculated that psychoses are caused by alterations of electrical activity in pathways connecting one or another of the projection fields with the center of ideas. Emil Kraepelin was initially attracted to Wernicke's theories but, when Wernicke failed to produce concrete evidence, Kraepelin turned against him. Nissl, too, rejected localization, at least with respect to mental illness. He believed that nerve cells, regardless of their locations, held the clues to mental illness. Critics began referring to Wernicke's ideas as "brain mythology".

Notwithstanding Wernicke's shortcomings, modern neuroscience has confirmed that in many respects function *is* localized in the brain. There is even evidence for partial localization of some mental illnesses. For example, brain correlates of schizophrenia seem especially prominent in the frontal lobe. Wernicke's theory of cerebral localization of function is still alive today, but it bears the scars of past battles.

–//–

Nerve cells, or neurons, were first seen in 1836. They were discovered by scientists practicing a particular sort of anatomy, that which concerns the structure of biological cells. These scientists are known as *histologists*. They slice up organic tissues, stain them, affix the sections to glass slides and examine them under microscopes. Gudden was an histologist, and so too was Nissl. The very early histologists had primitive microscopes and no means of coloring the tissues, so they saw only the largest cells, and these dimly. A breakthrough came when the histologists started staining their tissues with carmine, a powdery substance obtained from the female larvae of a scaly insect. It gave nerve cells a reddish color and made them and their nuclei stand out from the background.

A German histologist named Otto Deiters wanted to see even more, so he innovated. First, he used a special chemical solution that slightly hardened the brain. He sliced a thin section with a hand-held blade and stained the tissue with carmine dye. Finally, using a pair of fine needles, he gently teased out a single neuron from the surrounding tissue. It was micro-dissection, a tedious procedure that often failed, but when successful it enabled remarkably clear images of isolated neurons. Deiters had just enough time to draw a few highly accurate representations of those images before he died of typhoid fever at age twenty-nine. The drawings were published posthumously by his brother, in 1865.

Deiters' drawings show two types of delicate processes attached to the neuronal cell body (a particularly beautiful example adorns the cover of this book). The shorter processes, which he called protoplasmic extensions, are today known as dendrites, and they typically branch like a tree. Dendrites are specialized appendages that receive signals emitted by other neurons. Deiters called the longer, thicker processes axis cylinders, now known as axons. Usually each neuron has a single axon. Axons conduct electrical pulses from one neuron to another. They often gather together in the thousands or millions to form fiber bundles. Some bundles remain within the brain, while others become nerves, leaving the brain to connect with muscles and endocrine glands. Axons can be as short as a few micrometers or, in the case of axons that cause the toes to wriggle, about one meter long in an adult person of average height; the corresponding axons of a giraffe are much longer.

Deiters was not a psychiatrist, but a medical doctor with a small private practice. Most of his time was spent in the anatomy laboratory. Bernhard Gudden, by contrast was heavily involved in psychiatry, yet managed to conduct a substantial amount of neuroanatomical research "in his spare time", as the saying goes. Gudden's serious engagement with neuroanatomical research was directly inspired by Griesinger's call for a science-based psychiatry, so it is reasonable to ask, what was the nature of this research, and what were its results?

Anatomists had only a basic knowledge of the brain when Gudden began his research. They knew that it contained neurons, fibers and blood vessels. The neurons had various shapes. Some were roundish, some star-like, and still others pyramidal. Regardless of their types, the neurons tended to mass together in countless numbers, but never so tightly that individuals could not be discerned when using a high powered lens. The fibers were long and very thin and looked nothing like neurons. Individual fibers could be seen scattered around neurons, but they were most impressive when massed together in bundles, also known as tracts.

Finding cells in the brain did not surprise Gudden and colleagues, because Rudolf Virchow, student of Johannes Müller, had shown that cells are present everywhere in all plants and animals. But, their overwhelming numbers in the brain puzzled the neuroanatomists and raised many questions. Why are they unevenly distributed throughout the brain? Why do they appear in different sizes and different shapes? And, most obviously, what exactly do brain cells do, and how do they do it?

The fibrous structures raised other questions. The largest tracts, such as those crossing between the left and right hemispheres and those descending from the top of the brain down into the spinal cord, glisten white in freshly cut brains. They are obvious even to the naked eye. Because they span large distances and look much like nerves, they were understood to link different parts of the nervous system. More perplexing were the smaller fiber tracts. These, too, were thought to connect different parts of the brain, but it could not be determined which parts were connected to which other parts, because it was very difficult to trace them from their origins to their destinations. It was this problem of fiber pathways that Gudden tackled.

Sigmund Freud was one of the few histologists who had actually seen long fiber tracts in histological sections. He managed to do so by staining them with gold chloride. Other histologists used variants of Freud's gold chloride stain. The gold stains sometimes left fibers nicely colored in pink, purple, or blue, but more commonly they did not work at all. Later, it was discovered that hematoxylin, a substance obtained from logwood trees, worked much better. It stained nerve bundles darkly purple.

Gudden began his nerve fiber research in Zurich. He made his first discovery by examining brains with a simple magnifying glass. He noticed a fiber bundle running close to the optic tract at the back of the eye, but along the external surface of the brain. It diverges from the optic tract, crosses to the opposite side of the brain, and terminates at sites not visited by the optic tract. He called it the *tractus peduncularis transversus*. It forms part of what anatomists refer to as the accessory optic system, a group of fiber tracts that detects jittery visual images and helps to stabilize them in the "mind's eye". Gudden discovered the *tractus peduncularis transversus* while examining brains taken from rabbits. He subsequently found it in twelve more animal species as well as in humans. He also discovered another fiber tract, the supraoptic commissure, known today as Gudden's Commissure. Commissure is the anatomical term for a fiber tract that bridges the two halves of the brain. Gudden's Commissure passes directly over the optic nerves, but it has no function related to vision.

Also in Zurich, Gudden did an experiment with young rabbits demonstrating an important connection between the thalamus, a region near the center of the brain, and the cerebral cortex, the outermost shell of the brain. Gudden cut away part of the cortex and waited several weeks. When he then examined the brain, he noticed that some areas within the thalamus had shrunk. Looking more closely, he saw many dead or dying nerve cells. He correctly surmised that the damage he had inflicted on the cortex had spread to the thalamus along bands of fibers. It was the first evidence for what has since become a well-established fact, namely, that the thalamus relays motor and sensory signals to the cortex.

In Munich, Gudden put one of his assistant physicians, Dr. Sigbert Ganser, in charge of the neuroanatomy laboratory. Only a few of the research projects conducted there concerned human brains. Fewer still utilized the brains of psychiatric patients, and it was not for a lack of post-mortem material. The men were trying to learn about the basic composition and organization of vertebrate brains and, for this purpose, non-human animals offered certain advantages. Because they were smaller, they were easier to work with. Also, young animals could be used, and the histologists quickly found that staining was optimized in the immature nervous system. Fish, chickens, snakes, hedgehogs, moles and cats — all involuntarily gave up their brains for the advancement of science.

Gudden was fortunate in having easy access to the best microscopes in the world. They were manufactured by Ernst Leica in Wetzlar and Carl Zeiss in Jena, two companies that remain at the forefront of optical instrumentation today. He also had the latest photographic equipment. Still, Gudden faced formidable technical challenges. Even preparing brain tissues for microscopic examination was far from routine. Histologists needed to slice the brain into very thin sections. The slices had to be thin enough for light to penetrate through them, but not so thin as to wrinkle or break apart. As an approximation, they needed to be about fifty micrometers thick, or one-half the width of a human hair. It is impossible to slice a mushy brain so thinly.

To get around the problem, anatomists submersed the brain (or small pieces taken from it) into a solution of picric acid. After several days in the acid, the brain turned yellow, but the color was of no consequence. What mattered was that it was now hard enough to be cut with a sharp blade. The next problem was how to maneuver the blade so that it would cleanly slice off fifty micrometers, no more and no less. A mechanical device was needed, a sturdy instrument that could hold both the blade and the brain piece, then bring the two objects precisely together. In 1875, Gudden designed an instrument, a microtome, that was able to do that.

Gudden's microtome consisted of two moveable parts. The brain was affixed atop a metallic cylinder that could be moved up and down. A second device held the knife blade in such a manner that it could be slid through the brain. After cleaning the knife with alcohol, the microscopist submerged both the brain and the knife in water. He then raised, or lowered the brain piece until it appeared just slightly above the level of the knife; this was accomplished by turning a screw beneath the cylinder. Crucially, the thickness of the section could be finely and repeatedly adjusted, thanks to the precision of the screw mechanism. To cut sections, the knife was pushed along a rail until it passed through the tissue, allowing the detached section to float safely away. The section was picked up with a fine brush and placed on a glass microscope slide.

With the microtome now providing Gudden with a steady supply of high quality brain sections (he collected more than 50,000), he tackled the problem of fiber pathways within the brain. In principle, one could stain all the fibers with hematoxylin and then track a selected bundle as it moved through successive (serial) sections. Unfortunately, tracing a bundle of interest through a large number of brain sections can be a tedious and unrewarding task, because fibers typically traverse a dense jungle of cell bodies, dendrites and incidental nerve fibers en route to their destinations. Gudden invented a far more efficient method, based on his earlier work on thalamus-cortex connections. Now, instead of cutting away large areas of the cortex, he damaged the nerves associated with selected sense organs. After waiting for several weeks or months, he looked in the brain for degenerating axons, which had a very different appearance than intact, healthy fibers. Following these degenerating fibers, Gudden was able to reconstruct the pathways taken by the sensory nerves as they entered the brain.

Gudden used his new method to study the pathways taken by the optic nerves, a subject that had been debated for at least two hundred years. Each eye gives rise to its own optic nerve. There is a spot behind the eyes and centered between them where the two nerves appear to cross one another; it is called the optic chiasm. Some commentators interpreted this to mean that each eye sends its visual information to the opposite, or contralateral, side of the brain. To see if this was true, Gudden removed one eye from each of several young rabbits and young dogs. In every animal, he found that the optic nerves crossed *partially*, that is, some of the individual fibers in the each nerve went to the contralateral side while others stayed on the ipsilateral side. Later studies in humans demonstrated that about one-half of the fibers cross over. We get our binocular and stereoscopic vision from the partial crossing of the optic nerves.

Gudden made all of these discoveries, and more, while overseeing three hundred patients, a nursing staff and medical trainees at Munich's only mental hospital. Did his research benefit any of his patients? No, but his improvements to the microtome and his dogged pursuit of fiber pathways set an example for future psychiatrists determined to lay bare the brain's intricate structures. Although Gudden suffered an early death at Lake Starnberg, his neuroanatomical research remains alive in the scientific literature. Moreover, by putting into practice the hopeful message of Wilhelm Griesinger, Gudden made sure that his talented students would carry it even further.

After Gudden's death at Lake Starnberg, Franz Nissl followed up on his professor's work. Gudden had found – in his experiment linking the thalamus to the cortex – that nerve cell bodies shrivel up and die after their axons are damaged. He relied on the phenomenon to find the cells that give rise to the axon bundles that interested him. The cells died very slowly, however, after their axons were cut. Often the cell deaths could not be detected until weeks or months had passed. Nissl thought he might find a quicker, more reliable method.

There is a nerve, called the facial nerve, that runs from the brain to the face. Within this nerve lie thousands of axons, or fibers. They come from cells located somewhere in the brain. Where, exactly, are those cells?

Working with rabbits, Nissl located the facial nerve under the skin on its way from the brain to the face. He intentionally damaged it, then patched up the wound and waited a few days before killing the animal. He cut brain sections and stained them with methylene blue, an aniline dye. Next, Nissl scanned slide after slide until he found what he was looking for. Deep in the brainstem, near the spinal cord, he noticed a group of neurons whose nuclei were exceptionally dark and displaced to the edges of the cell. Also, the granules that he had discovered during his student days in Munich were broken up and barely recognizable, in contrast to nearby neurons in which the granules looked normal. Nissl surmised that the cells with the dark, displaced nuclei and the broken-up granules had axons in the nerve that he damaged. These axons, from those cells, formed the facial nerve.

Here was a method for tracing fiber pathways that was quicker and easier than Gudden's. It would be used not just for finding the origins of nerves, but also for discovering connections between one area of the brain and another. Knowledge of that sort was needed to resolve issues around the hypothesized localization of function. For example, it had been proposed that conduction aphasia might be caused by a disconnection between the brain area responsible for speech comprehension (Wernicke's area) and the area responsible for speech production (Broca's area). Obviously, for there to be such a disconnection, the connection itself must first be confirmed in undamaged brains. Later research demonstrated that, in fact, there is no such connection.

11 Seeing is Believing, or Maybe Not

Nissl and his fellow histologists were familiar with the various sizes and shapes of neurons. What they did not understand, and what puzzled them, was the anatomical relationship between individual neurons. It was a daunting problem. Does each neuron stand as an independent unit or do neurons connect to one another through their axons? The fiber bundles studied by Gudden and Nissl are made of axons. They originate at neuronal cell bodies, but what becomes of them at their endings? Does the axon of one neuron fuse with the axon of another neuron? Does it fuse with another cell body, with dendrites, or with nothing at all? Histologists needed to know whether or not neurons are connected through fibrous linkages, and to find out, they needed a method that would clearly reveal axon endings. But there were none. In the eyes of *some* microscopists, looking at *some* examples, the axons *appeared* to contact cell dendrites. Other axons *appeared* to contact cell bodies. The microscopic images were too fuzzy for anyone to be sure.

In the absence of hard facts, neuroanatomists throughout Europe took sides. Those who thought that the nervous system is a collection of individual cells standing alone, in other words, *not* fusing, were called neuronists. In the opposite camp were the reticularists, named after the reticulum, or web, that they thought connected the neurons. Albert von Kölliker was a respected anatomist and also a reticularist. His drawing, published in 1867, illustrates a reticularist's conception of the nervous system (Figure 19). Note that all the structures are shown fused together. It must be emphasized that the drawing is schematic; it depicts what Kölliker *imagined*, not what he actually *saw*.

The controversy about neurons and nerve nets had no direct bearing on mental illness, yet many of the anatomists participating in the debate were psychiatrists. Why? Because they understood that knowing whether the brain is a reticulum or a collection of individual cells is essential to understanding how the brain works, and knowing how it works is a precondition for knowing how it malfunctions.

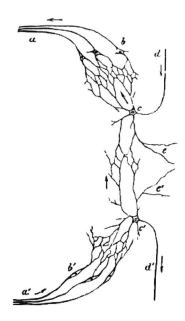

Figure 19: The nervous system depicted as a web of connected structures. The labelled structures *b*, *b'*, *c* and *c'* are nerve cells; *a* and *d* are axons. The unlabeled, branched structures are dendrites. [Albert von Kölliker, 1867]

One of the histologists competing to resolve the issue of reticulum versus neuronism was Joseph von Gerlach, who invented a staining method for just that purpose. After viewing sections stained with the new method, Gerlach declared, "I have been able to show with the gold method the *continuity* [italics added] of the network [axons] with the protoplasmic prolongations [dendrites] of the nerve cells."[79] In other words, he had found evidence to support the reticular theory – or so he believed.

In Italy, Camillo Golgi from the University of Pavia, was also working on a new staining method. His method was much better than Gerlach's, and good enough for a Nobel Prize. Golgi hardened his sections in a solution made of potassium bichromate and osmic acid. He then immersed the sections in a dilute solution of silver nitrate. The resulting silver-chromate precipitate made the neurons appear black. Whereas the carmine and aniline dyes used by Nissl and his German colleagues stained the nerve cell

---

[79]Quoted in Gordon M. Shepherd, *Foundations of the Neuron Doctrine*, 25th anniversary ed., New York, Oxford University Press (2016), p. 57.

bodies, and only the bodies, the silver method revealed all parts of the neurons. Crucially, the silver stain showed the delicate dendritic branches and the fine fibers in exquisite detail. Only about one in ten neurons took up the silver –for unknown reasons – but this was actually a good thing, because it allowed every stained neuron to be viewed in its entirety. If all neurons were stained equally well, the whole slide would be blackened, making it impossible to see anything well.

In a report published in 1873, Golgi claimed that he saw fused fibers. In his words, "It being demonstrated ... that a nervous fibre is in relation with extensive groups of ganglia cells [neurons], and that the gangliar elements of entire provinces, and also of various neighboring provinces, are conjoined by means of a diffuse network ... it is naturally difficult [in light of the foregoing] to understand a rigorous functional localization, as many would have it."[80] Golgi was thinking of Wernicke, whose localization theory Golgi disliked.

Franz Nissl was also in the reticularist camp, even though the staining techniques at his disposal (aniline dyes) precluded him from personally confirming (or refuting) their claims. He, Golgi and many others, felt that the reticular idea must be right because localization was wrong. If functions are distributed rather than localized, then the brain must be a continuous web rather than a collection of solitary neurons.

Lining up on the side of the neuronists were Otto Deiters, August Forel (an accomplished anatomist and former student of Wilhelm Gudden) and several other reputable German microscopists. Deiters had reported certain observations that seemed to show gaps between axons and dendrites – rather than the continuity claimed by Gerlach and Golgi – but the evidence remained inconclusive at the time of his early death.

Also weighing in on the issue was Sigmund Freud, in Vienna. Before practicing psychotherapy – even before working as a neuropathologist (and writing about aphasia) – he did neuroanatomical research at the Physiological Institute in Vienna. The work ranged from studies of invertebrate nervous systems to studies of the human brain. He published several papers on staining methods and another on the structure of neurons and nerve fibers in crayfish. In 1884, he gave a lecture before the Viennese Psychiatric Society in which he addressed, among other things, the question of cellular organization in the nervous system. Freud said (as it was later reported),

---

[80]G. M. Shepherd (2016), p. 94.

> [I]f ... the fibrils of the nerve fiber have the function of isolated
> conductive pathways [which] are confluent in the nerve cell, the
> nerve cell becomes the beginning of all those nerve fibers which
> are anatomically connected to it ... Then we could consider the
> possibility that the nerve as a unit conducts the excitation.[81]

In stating that nerve fibers (axons) are "confluent in" (emanate from) nerve cells, and in suggesting that nerve cells act as units, Freud's thoughts echoed those of the neuronists.

In October of 1889, neuronists and reticularists gathered in Berlin for a meeting of the German Anatomical Society. The event was hosted by Wilhelm von Waldeyer-Hartz, then head of the Anatomy Department at the University of Berlin. His distinguished reputation, along with the prestige of the Anatomical Society, ensured a good attendance. Men (again, only men) from Norway, Sweden, Belgium, Spain and all parts of Germany came to the event. In comparison to modern neuroscience conventions at which attendances can reach over 30,000, the total number of attendees at the Berlin meeting was miniscule. Nevertheless, in the two rooms given over to the meeting, the air was hot with anticipation and thick with cigar smoke. The meeting marked a turning point in the history of neuroscience because, for the first time, the microscope slides of a previously obscure Spanish anatomist were seen by scientists outside his home country.

Santiago Ramón y Cajal, the anatomist with the splendid slides, provided a vivid description of the Berlin conference in his delightful autobiography.[82] The young scientist prepared for his first trip to Germany knowing full well that he would find in Berlin many of the anatomists whose work he had read about and emulated. "I gathered together for the purpose all my scanty savings and set out, full of hope for the capital of the German Empire." Upon arriving in Berlin, he was pleased by the "courteous" reception accorded him by his colleagues. As for the colleagues' reaction to him – the stranger from afar – he wrote, "It was a shock for them, no doubt, to meet a Spaniard who cultivated science and had of his own volition entered upon the paths of research." Not only had the Germans never encountered a Spaniard at any of their meetings, Cajal was a different sort of scientist. Born of humble origins in the district of Aragon in

---

[81] Quote from L. C. Triarhou and M. del Cerro, "Freud's contribution to neuroanatomy," *Archives of Neurology* 42:282-287 (1985).

[82] Santiago Ramón y Cajal, *Recollections of My Life*, translated by E. Horne Craigie, Cambridge, MA, M.I.T Press (1937). The account of the Berlin conference is on pages 355-359.

northeastern Spain, he had labored for years in nearly complete isolation. His passion for neuroanatomy, however, was no less intense than that of his northern counterparts. Only thirty-seven years of age at the time of the Berlin meeting, he had penetrating eyes, a long straight nose and a neatly trimmed, dark beard. He neither smoked nor drank alcohol. No one could have mistaken him for a German.

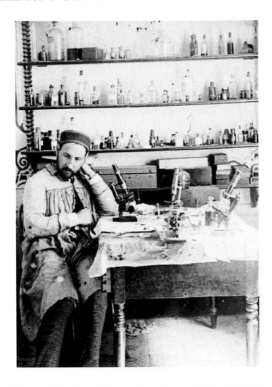

Figure 20: Santiago Ramón y Cajal, 1887.

Cajal sat impatiently through the first event of the conference, the oral presentations. He knew little German and was, in any case anxiously awaiting the start of the next event, the demonstrations. Traveling by train from Barcelona, he had brought with him his precious Zeiss microscope. During a break between the oral presentations and the demonstrations, Cajal placed the microscope on a table in the demonstration room, and he set up three locally requisitioned microscopes in a similar manner. Next, he removed his four best glass slides from a small, well cushioned box and put one slide under each microscope. Finally, he precisely positioned each slide so that the microscope lens bore directly down on its best features.

With these four slides, and others retained in the small box, Cajal meant to demonstrate the power of Golgi's silver staining method. He had modified the method by cutting thicker sections and adding a second round of hardening followed by a second immersion in silver. The thicker sections allowed a microscopist to see all parts of the stained neurons by focusing up and down within the section. The added cycles of hardening and staining produced a darker stain. As well, Cajal used very young animals for his studies, again because the stain worked best in these animals. The slides that he brought to Berlin showcased neurons and fibers from many different areas of the nervous system including the cerebrum, the cerebellum, the retina and the spinal cord.

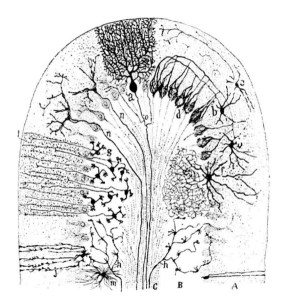

Figure 21: Cajal's drawing of neuron types in the mammalian cerebellum, from silver stained tissue sections. Schematic presentation combining observations from numerous individual sections.

Never before had Cajal's northern colleagues seen silver-stained neurons. "[T]hese savants, then world celebrities, began their examination with more skepticism than curiosity. Undoubtedly, they expected a fiasco. However, when there had been paraded before their eyes in a procession of irreproachable images of the utmost clearness ... the supercilious frowns disappeared."

Obviously, Cajal had moved beyond his humble beginnings by the time of writing his autobiography.

Along with his slides, Cajal brought strong reasons for rejecting reticularism and accepting neuronism. The general argument was three-fold. First, where the slides showed immature neurons growing in embryonic brains, no part of any neuron was seen touching any other neuron or any fiber. Second, damaged neurons were seen degenerating as single units, leaving neighboring cells unaffected. Third, where axons approached a neuronal cell body or one of its dendrites, small gaps could be seen between the fiber endings and the cell body or dendrite. Ironically, the last mentioned observation turned out to be an artifact of Cajal's staining procedure, but in the end it did not matter, because synapses, which are the definitive proof of the gaps between neurons, were discovered in 1955 using an electron microscope. While Cajal's arguments were mostly technical, he also noted the distressing implications of the reticular theory, "To affirm that everything communicates with everything else is equivalent to declaring the absolute unsearchability of the organ of the soul."[83]

There can be no doubt about the effects of Cajal's demonstrations on the "savants". Albert von Kölliker, whom Cajal described as the "venerable patriarch of German histology", took special notice. As noted above, Kölliker was a backer of reticularism, or at least he was until he met Cajal and viewed his slides. He befriended Cajal, taught himself Spanish so he could read Cajal's papers, and persuaded Cajal to give him detailed instructions for silver-staining. In the ensuing years, Kölliker replicated many of Cajal's most controversial findings. He rejected net theory and joined the neuronist camp. Wilhelm Waldeyer-Hartz, host of the Berlin conference, also learned Spanish so that he could fully absorb Cajal's arguments. Although he did not contribute new histological work, Waldeyer-Hartz wrote a lengthy defense of the neuron theory that brought many anatomists to Cajal's side. In the course of writing the article, Waldeyer-Hartz coined the term "neuron".

Santiago Ramón y Cajal and Camillo Golgi were jointly awarded Nobel prizes in 1906 for their ground breaking work, even though Golgi was not yet convinced of the neuron theory. To this day, Cajal's drawings continue to draw admiration from practicing neuroscientists, and his life story serves as an inspiration for all kinds of scientists. Buried in the middle of his autobiography is a short paragraph, written in his inimitable style, that speaks to the passionate character of this remarkable man,

---

[83]S. R. Y. Cajal (1937), p. 338.

It is an actual fact that, leaving aside the flatteries of self-love, the garden of neurology holds out to the investigator captivating spectacles and incomparable artistic emotions. In it my aesthetic instincts found full satisfaction at last. Like the entomologist in pursuit of brightly colored butterflies, my attention hunted, in the flower garden of the gray matter [the cerebrum], cells with delicate and elegant forms, the mysterious butterflies of the soul the beating of whose wings may some day – who knows? – clarify the secret of mental life.[84]

Franz Nissl probably attended the Berlin conference in 1889, although no record confirms it. Assuming that he did attend, we can further assume that he presented his recent work on progressive paralysis, research that was conducted in collaboration with Alois Alzheimer. He probably gave a talk about the work, wearing his customarily disheveled clothing and speaking in his rambling, ungrammatical manner. After the talk, he would have demonstrated slides showing the cellular deformations and blood vessel aberrations characteristic of the illness. His colleagues, who generally appreciated his open personality and quirky sense of humor, would have applauded politely. Nevertheless, Nissl must have felt sidelined at the Berlin conference (assuming his presence), because the buzz was about Cajal's gorgeous black neurons and their important implications. Nissl had little to contribute to the debate over reticularism and neuronism because he was a specialist in the use of aniline dyes, and they did not stain fibers. If he ever tried using the Golgi-Cajal silver stain, there is nothing in his writings to suggest that it worked for him.

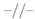

Because Nissl was an anatomist *and* a psychiatrist he appreciated the fact that the brain is not just an organ for controlling facial movements, it is also – most probably – home to the mind. Or was it the soul? He struggled to understand how the soul differs from the mind, and where the brain fits in. Although his father had tried to steer him into the priesthood, Nissl was not a religious man. In spite of that, he occasionally welcomed into his Heidelberg apartment the parish priest from his hometown, whom he had known since his youth. There is no record of what was said in those meetings, but one can imagine Nissl inquiring about the soul. What,

---

[84]S. R. Y. Cajal (1937), p. 363.

exactly, is it? And where, exactly, does it reside? Philosophers have tripped over the same questions for millennia. Indeed, we all do. Maybe the priest suggested some answers that Nissl found useful. But Nissl, the scientist, must have wanted more. Understandably, therefore, he grew feverish with excitement when he learned of an anatomical finding that possibly held the key to all of this.

Nissl's interest was aroused by research that was being done at the Zoological Laboratory in Naples, Italy, by a Hungarian scientist named Stephan von Apáthy. Histologists were always hoping to find structures never seen before and, as readers of this book may have gathered by now, the most common route to a new observation was the invention of a better stain. In Apáthy's case, his breakthrough discovery came after he incorporated gold chloride into the hardening solution, similar to what Freud and Gerlach had done.

The novel structures revealed by Apáthy's stain were very thin fibers, known as fibrils. They were violet in color and much finer than any of the axons or dendrites seen by other histologists. According to Apáthy's description, the fibrils formed a diffuse web all around the neurons, and some passed right through cells. Apáthy interpreted the fibrils as conducting elements, meaning he thought they conveyed information from one neuron to another. In effect, he was reporting new evidence in favor of the reticulum theory of cellular organization.

Nissl was initially skeptical. After all, the fibrils had only been observed in a marine leech, not in any animal possessed of a backbone. While he subscribed to Charles Darwin's theory of evolution, he was not prepared to accept findings from a leech as evidence that fibrils are present in the human brain. But then Nissl read that Albrecht Bethe, a German physiologist and anatomist, had found fibrils in vertebrate brains. The news persuaded Nissl that fibrils were real – and very interesting.

Nissl's own work was still focused on nerve cell bodies, they being the objects best stained by aniline dyes. He had enjoyed early success with the discovery of tiny granules (the eponymous Nissl bodies), and his work with Alzheimer on progressive paralysis had been well received. So, too, was he getting credit from peers for his method of tracing fiber pathways by examining cell body structures. Other projects, however had not turned out so well. With the exception of progressive paralysis, he had not found strong evidence of neuropathology in any mental illness. Now, the reports of Apáthy and Bethe gave him pause to reconsider. Perhaps nerve cells, that is nerve cell *bodies*, were not really so important. Maybe they were not responsible for the brain's functions. Maybe Apáthy's fibrils held the key to understanding the brain.

As Nissl arrived in Baden for the twenty-third meeting of the Association of Southwest German Neurologists and Psychiatrists (commonly known as the Hiking Meeting), he anticipated that his colleagues would want to hear about his most recent research. That work, on using drugs to model mental illness, had not gone well, as will become apparent below. So, when it came time for Nissl to speak, he briefly summarized that failed research and then quickly turned to the work of Apáthy and Bethe. Because he was speaking before a sympathetic audience comprised mostly of friends and collaborators, he felt no restraint in presenting the unconventional conclusions that he had drawn from Apáthy's discovery. As he warmed to the task, his voice grew louder, his speech more rapid, and his sense more muddled.[85]

He asked his esteemed colleagues to imagine two components in the nervous system. First, he said, the familiar nerve cell. Second, a substance fundamentally different from any cell, fiber, or other structure in the brain, but present everywhere. He called this substance "gray matter", and he acknowledged Apáthy's role in discovering the interwoven mass of fine fibrils from which his concept derived. He repeatedly stated that the true nature of the gray matter is unknown. Regardless, he asserted that the real work of the nervous system is done not by nerve cells, but by gray matter.

As proof of his contention, Nissl offered two lines of evidence. The first came from work done by Albrecht Bethe at the Naples Zoological Laboratory. Bethe's attention had been drawn to the antennae of some local crabs. The antennae are long, paired appendages that move about in the water sensing chemicals and hard surfaces. When Bethe found fibrils inside the antennae, he decided to conduct an experiment. He painstakingly removed all the nerve cells – but none of the fibrils – from the antennae of several crabs. After the animals recovered from the surgery, he tested their reflexes by touching their antennae. Healthy crabs rapidly withdraw their antennae at the slightest touch, and the experimental animals did that too. Since all the nerve cells had been removed from the antenna of the experimental crabs, it was clearly the fibrils, not the nerve cells, that were responsible for the movements.

---

[85]Nissl's address at the meeting of the *Versammlung der Südwestdetuschen Neurologen und Irrenärtze*, in Baden, was published in the *Münchener Medicinische Wochenschrift*, pp. 988-1063 (1898).

The second proof came from Nissl's own examination of the cerebrum in three mammalian species: moles, dogs and humans. In this investigation, he looked only at the spaces between nerve cells, guided by the following reasoning. Assuming that gray matter – invisible with his methods – was filling the space between the cells, he expected to see the largest spaces in humans, somewhat smaller spaces in dogs, and the smallest in moles, because the more "advanced" the species, the more gray matter it should have. Sure enough, that is exactly what he found. The anatomical results, he told his audience in Baden, correlated perfectly with the intelligence of the species. Hearing this, the neurologists and psychiatrists of southwestern Germany may have squirmed and fiddled in their seats, but they waited to hear more.

Nissl's voice became even more animated, his language more fractured, as he broadened his message. He stated his belief that the advanced animal species need something more than nerve cells – more, indeed, than *all* types of cells – to support their functions. That additional something was gray matter. He explained,

> From this point of view, the idea, somewhat strange to our usual thought, becomes intelligible, that the highest functions of the vertebrate body are not directly attached to cells, but to a living substance, the morphological arrangement of which reminds one much rather of anything else than of cells. We need only look carefully into our body to convince ourselves readily that the most differentiated sense-organs, or the voluntary muscles, offer similar relations.

What, then, is the function of nerve cells?

> The cells play a role in the nervous system, but they are not responsible for its functions. Rather, it is the gray matter, distinct from the cells, that controls our thoughts and actions. Although we do not yet know the true essence of the gray matter, it is the most highly evolved protoplasm[86] in the entire body. For these

---

[86]Protoplasm is an older term roughly corresponding to the modern term, cytoplasm. In the late nineteenth century, it was widely believed that protoplasm was the fundamental substance of life.

reasons, you will surely agree with me that the neuron theory cannot be correct.[87]

So there it was, Nissl's ultimate refutation of neuronism. The presentation drew a mixed reception from the assembled doctors. Some men were impressed, but most were simply confused. The American psychiatrist Adolph Meyer later wrote that the speech was "long and not lucid." Meyer had recently spent six weeks visiting Kraepelin and Nissl in Heidelberg. Upon returning to America, Meyer became (for a short while) an enthusiastic supporter of Kraepelin's brand of psychiatry. Nevertheless, his criticism of Nissl's radical ideas was scathing.

> Many expressions [were] given meanings which seem to be the fountain-head of confusion; I mention only his use of the term 'cell'. Nissl's cell is a decidedly expurgated affair, a sponge through the holes of which the 'real nervous substance' grows quite irrespective of the fact that the fibrils and expurgated cell-concept are together that which we are accustomed to call cell for reasons too simple to be offered to Dr. Nissl. The same holds for 'gray matter' of which nobody would ever think that it meant what Nissl wants it to mean. Perhaps this terminology is necessary to produce the degree of obscurity so popular for certain kinds of demonstrations.[88]

Moreover, many persons in attendance at the Baden meeting firmly believed in the neuron theory. They knew and respected Albert von Kölliker, who was by now championing that theory, and some had even read Ramón y Cajal's articles. One imagines that the men gave Nissl a round of applause for his provocative presentation, and immediately filed out of the lecture hall for supper. Gray matter had had its day, but it was a short day.

Nissl made a big deal out of fibrils, and it turned out that he was wrong to do so. That does not make him a bad scientist. It only means that in this particular instance, his enthusiasm was misplaced. As a rule, science needs

---

[87] The quoted passages from Nissl's lecture were translated into English by Adolph Meyer, "Critical review of recent publications of Bethe and Nissl," *Journal of Comparative Neurology* 9:38-45 (1899).

[88] A. Meyer (1898), p. 43. Nissl's concept of gray matter differs from current usage, where gray matter refers to the cell-rich regions of the cerebral cortex, contrasting to the fiber-rich regions known as white matter.

bold ideas. If proven false, they can be forgotten, but when proven true, they jumpstart new inventions and new medical advances. As for the fibrils first described by Apáthy and Bethe, they are now known to constitute the neuron's cytoskeleton, a network of protein filaments that maintains the cell's structural integrity. All types of cells, not just neurons, have cytoskeletons. Unfortunately, Nissl thought they had an entirely different function.

12 Mind-Altering Drugs and Disease-Causing Poisons

Drugs were everywhere, it seems, in nineteenth century psychiatry. Ubiquitous in clinical wards, they were also present in research laboratories. Like now, they were usually beneficial when taken for medical purposes, and generally benign when used cautiously for recreational purposes, but toxic or poisonous when taken in high dosages. Nineteenth century psychiatrists were well aware of this dual character. They both feared it and exploited it.

Psychiatrists knew that certain drugs are mentally destabilizing, and can cause serious mental derangements in susceptible individuals. Based on those observations, they hypothesized that at least some mental illnesses might be caused by unidentified substances acting as poisons in the human body. Both ingested poisons and internally produced substances were suspect. During the last half of the nineteenth century, marijuana was hardly known, cocaine was rare, and few of the prescription drugs familiar to us today existed. The dominate drug, by far, was alcohol, and it is the perfect example of a drug that was capable of multiple effects, both good and bad. It was at once a social lubricant, a medication and a deadly poison. As such, it will be given special treatment later in this chapter.

The drug most commonly used in asylums and clinics was chloral hydrate. It was one of several compounds known as "hypnotics" due to their ability to sedate patients and put them to sleep. Chloral hydrate was particularly effective, but also addictive and toxic. First synthesized in 1832 (by the chlorination of alcohol), it was not used as a medicine until 1869. Thereafter, chloral hydrate quickly found a place in psychiatric practice. Two additional synthetic drugs, sulphonal and the faster-acting trional, came on the scene somewhat later. Hyoscyamine and hyoscine were both extracted from nightshade plants; they were cheaper than choral hydrate, but less potent. Potassium bromide was the cheapest of all the hypnotic drugs, but it had to used cautiously because it induced nausea, vomiting and even seizures. The main non-sedating medications were urethane (ethyl carbamate) and alcohol, the latter used primarily with depressed or mildly agitated patients. Highly agitated patients were given morphine. The drug of choice for any particular patient depended on its availability and cost, in addition to the experience of the prescribing doctor.

Long before the use of sedatives became commonplace, Hippocrates and his fellow physicians treated mentally disturbed patients with purgatives. Hippocrates believed that all disorders, both physical and mental, were caused by the excessive accumulation of certain substances in the human body, which he called humors. Therefore, to purge his patients of a harmful humor, he gave them powders made from the roots of the black Hellebore plant. Hippocrates observed that Hellebore induces a kind of hysterical suffocation in women, along with menstruation and vomiting. He imagined that the blood and vomit removed the offending humor from the body.

Bloodletting was another way of ridding the body of poisonous substances. Already used by physicians in ancient Greece, its popularity increased even more after the highly reputed Galen promoted it in the second century AD. In the late seventeenth century, Thomas Willis, the otherwise wise physician and accomplished neuroanatomist, practiced bloodletting. Even at the end of the eighteenth century, venesection, or the cutting of veins, was commonly employed in French asylums, although Phillipe Pinel denounced it. And finally, doctors applied leeches to the patients' skin so that the animals could suck out the bad blood.

The notion that bad things happen after bad things enter the body became all the more real after Louis Pasteur and Robert Koch discovered those microscopic organisms called germs. Psychiatrists combined the new germ theory of physical disease with the earlier notion of drug toxicity to forge a new hypothesis for mental diseases. They imagined bacteria breaking down tissue proteins, which would then release toxic residues into the blood. The toxins were thought to affect mental health indirectly by disrupting the secretion of natural substances, primarily hormones. In the final step, the hormonal imbalance affected brain activity. It was an idea built in part on Griesinger's theory of mental reflexes, wherein mental illness were caused by either insufficient activity or excessive activity.

Evidence for the role of hormonal imbalance came from the example of myxedema, which is a serious disease manifested by multiple symptoms. Of particular interest, is its association with a form of psychosis known as myxedema madness. Myxedema was thought to be caused by a deficiency of thyroid hormone, and an English physician proved that to be true by successfully treating a patient with an extract made from a sheep's thyroid gland.

Spurred by these developments, Nissl became interested in studying the cerebrospinal fluid, which is a clear, colorless fluid that bathes the brain and spinal cord. Although the cerebrospinal fluid is now understood to act primarily as a physical cushion, little was known about it in Nissl's time. His mind was drawn to the possibility that the cerebrospinal fluid could become contaminated. If so, it might hold clues to mental illness. So Nissl started thinking that there might be something of interest in the chemistry of the cerebrospinal fluid. When word of a new medical procedure come to his attention, he saw his opportunity to test the idea. He learned of the procedure from the published report of a medical meeting held in the town of Wiesbaden in 1891.

A local doctor named Heinrich Quincke had been studying the circulation of the cerebrospinal fluid in dogs. His method consisted of releasing a bit of dye into the cerebrospinal fluid from a needle inserted between two spinal bones. This allowed him to watch as the colored patch of cerebrospinal fluid moved its way through the nervous system. At around the same time as Quincke was conducting these experiments, he became aware of some cases of childhood hydrocephalus, a serious medical condition caused by excessive fluids in the brain. The worst affected children suffered terrible headaches and had noticeably swollen heads. Quincke thought that if he could relieve pressure in the brain by withdrawing cerebrospinal fluid, he might cure the condition. Experimenting with one patient, he inserted a long needle between two of the child's spinal bones – as he had done with his dogs – but instead of injecting dye, he withdrew fluid. The treatment did not work, but it drew the attention of Nissl, who soon became smitten with spinal puncture.

At Heidelberg, Nissl copied Quincke's techniques. Over the course of many years, he withdrew cerebrospinal fluid from hundreds of patients. He did not find any substances in the fluid relevant to psychiatric illness, but he did develop a method for quantifying the fluid's protein content, and modern versions of that method are used today in psychiatric research. Nissl's students were so impressed with his frequent demonstrations of spinal puncture, they gave him the nickname, *Punctator Maximus*.

$$-//-$$

We do not know what particular substances Nissl was looking for in the cerebrospinal fluid, but he most likely viewed them as poisons, because he believed that it was poisons of one sort or another that cause mental illness. In further pursuit of the hypothesis, he launched an experimental test. He did it in a roundabout way by studying brain cells instead of mental illness, and using rabbits instead of humans as his subjects. The rationale linking poisons, rabbit brain cells and mental illness is a bit complicated, so I will explain.

Nissl thought that there were five types of neurons in the cerebral cortex, based on the structures seen within their cell bodies. (Today, hundreds of neuron types are recognized, based mostly on biochemical, electrophysiological and anatomical criteria. See Figure 21 on page 132.) Nissl identified one type in which the cytoplasm (the non-nuclear portion the cell interior) was completely unstained, while the nucleus was heavily stained and unusually large. Another type had a small, lightly stained nucleus. The remaining types were distinguished by the size and arrangement of the dark granules that he had discovered in Munich.

Neuron types were important for Nissl, and he believed that each type had a unique function. He did not elaborate on these functions, but one can imagine that they might govern such things as movement, mood, volition and intelligence.

The relationship between neuron types and mental illness, according to Nissl, was quite simple. He assumed, first of all, that nerve cell abnormalities could explain all forms of mental illness. Further, he assumed that the type of illness depended on which type of neuron was abnormal. So, for example, mental disorder type A might be caused by abnormalities in neuron type Y whereas mental disorder type B would be due to abnormalities in neuron type Z. It was the hypothesis that drove his work with Alzheimer on progressive paralysis. That research was successful in that neuronal pathologies were found, but it also disappointed Nissl because those pathologies were present not in any single cell type, but rather, in *all* cell types.

Still, Nissl was not ready to give up on the idea. Maybe progressive paralysis was special, or maybe he and Alzheimer had not carried out the investigation in the best possible manner. He thought about poisons. If poisons were responsible for mental illnesses, then different poisons should cause different mental disorders by affecting different types of neurons. This cell-based theory was Nissl's answer to Wernicke's location-based theory.

To test the theory, Nissl injected rabbits with a single strong dose of a commonly available drug such as morphine, tetanus toxin, or strychnine. After waiting several weeks, he killed the animals, cut their brains into sections and stained with methylene blue dye. As anticipated, he found odd-appearing structures inside some of the neurons. However, he had to look hard to find good examples, and he could not determine whether each poison produced a specific type of change in a specific type of cell. So, he altered the experiment. Instead of administering just a single dose of the poison, he injected many weaker doses over the course of several weeks or months. One particular rabbit received a small dose of morphine every day for nine months. When Nissl looked at these brains, he saw more instances of cellular pathology, but to his dismay, there were absolutely no correlations between poisons and affected cell types.

Experiments fail for many reasons. The research animals can be sick, the equipment defective, the sampling biased, or the environment surrounding the experiment uncontrolled. It is also possible for an investigator to err in his execution of the experiment or in the analysis of its results. Nissl had many research disappointments, and he usually attributed his failures to the last mentioned cause. In the case of the poisoning experiments, however, he had to admit that the ideas that motivated the experiments were wrong. He was forced to abandon the twined hypotheses of toxic causes and function-specific neuron types. It was with these disappointments still fresh in his mind that he traveled to Baden for the meeting of neurologists and psychiatrists, the meeting at which he spoke so passionately about gray matter.

Fortunately, the self-doubt and self-incrimination so characteristic of Nissl's personality was matched by an ability to rebound from failures. Time and time again, he was saved from despair by a wellspring of fresh ideas. After conceding defeat with the poisoning experiments, for example, he managed to move forward thanks to the epiphany on gray matter. And even after that disaster, there were still more ideas yet to be tested.

$$-//-$$

Alcohol is a drug of special interest. In the beginning, when societies were rural and mostly agrarian, it was woven into the normal fabric of life. Then industrialization created a disadvantaged social class that tended to drink excessively. The problem arose first in England, then spread to the continent. When politicians and social commentators became concerned, so too did Benedict Morel and Henry Maudsley, who promptly came up with degeneration theory to explain the association between class and alcohol (see Chapter 3).

In reality, the relationship between alcohol and industrialization was complex. Certainly, alcohol aggravated labor-management relations in the latter half of the nineteenth century. Workers were being asked to perform unaccustomed tasks and give up entrenched habits. Many responded to the pressure by taking to the bottle. According to one contemporary account, alcohol was a constant feature at German construction sites in the 1870s,

> *Schnaps* [a fruit-flavored alcoholic drink] had to be fetched on every occasion; when a new journeyman started work, for example, he was obliged first to provide a liter of *Schnaps* as his initiation. When an apprentice completed his first corner or curve, he too had to produce a liter of *Schnaps* for others. And so it went.[89]

Management, on the other hand, demanded efficiency and compliance. A German economist and philanthropist reported that

> drinkers are useless for industrial purposes: they quickly become sluggish, are slow on the job, unreliable, contentious, prone to frequent illness and, in the long run, impossible to protect against the dangers of machine production ... They must be dismissed from the job and replaced by sober hands [note 90].

All the problems surrounding alcohol got wrapped up in what became known as the "drink question". Actually, there were numerous questions. Is drinking ruining the economy? Is drinking good – or bad – for peoples' health? Is it natural or is it immoral? And, does it mix well with politics? Only the last question was easily answered. European socialists, including Karl Marx and Frederick Engels, defended the workers' right to drink, claiming it as a necessary response to capitalist pressures. Others, turned off by what they perceived as the offensive and threatening atmosphere in beer halls, where socialist groups tended to meet, joined temperance movements. So no, alcohol and politics did not mix well.

Beer was the most popular alcoholic drink in Germany. The German Purity Law (*Reinheitsgebot*), promulgated in Bavaria in 1516, was largely responsible. It was originally designed to prevent competition between brewers and bakers over the price of grains that were used in both crafts. But it also prevented the importation of northern beers into the Bavarian market. With time, once the Purity Law had spread to all German states, it became an effective non-tariff barrier to foreign competition. German breweries grew and prospered. In the 1880s, Germany surpassed Britain as the world's leading consumer.

---

[89]Quotes from James S. Roberts, "Drink and industrial work discipline in 19th century Germany," *Journal of Social History* 15: 25-38 (1981).

Physicians began calling attention to alcohol's deleterious effects. They saw heavy drinkers develop liver damage and delirium tremens, the latter a serious condition involving tremors, hallucinations and mental confusion. Gustav Aschaffenburg, Kraepelin's assistant physician in Heidelberg, wrote his dissertation on delirium tremens. It was a technical work that found only a small, professional readership. By contrast, another book on the medical consequences of alcoholic consumption, by the Swedish physician Magnus Huss, had a huge impact. Huss complied and assessed a mass of information on the unhealthy effects of alcohol. From these data, he concluded that people who drink heavily are truly sick, and he named the illness "alcoholism". Huss's book, published in 1849, marked a turning point in attitudes toward alcohol. It initiated the temperance movement, and it engaged the medical/scientific community as never before.

The Good Templars organization was founded in the United States in 1851 with the goal of improving society by limiting the use of alcohol. Similar movement sprang up in Europe and beyond. The first of several international congresses was held in Antwerp in 1885. By the mid-1880s, the German Society Opposed to the Abuse of Spirituous Liquors was arguing for changes to licensing laws and calling for the medical treatment of alcohol abusers.

–//–

Meanwhile, alcohol was being given to psychiatric patients to calm their nerves and encourage their sleep. Kraepelin used it for that purpose. He also occasionally gave it to patients suffering from obsessions, melancholia, or agoraphobia (anxieties related to open or crowded spaces) – not as a cure, but rather as something that could boost their self-confidence and temporarily lessen their suffering. He also used alcohol in his pharmacopsychological investigations. Recall that he studied the effect of alcohol on reaction times when he was with Wilhelm Wundt in Leipzig. Later, in Dorpat, he conducted numerous, separate investigations of the effects of alcohol on verbal associations, reading, serial addition, number learning, dynamometer (force) associations and time estimations. He obtained results, but as in Leipzig, the data were inconsistent and difficult to interpret.

With time, Kraepelin became more and more concerned about the negative effects of alcohol. As a first step, he prohibited its use in the clinic. Then he, himself, stopped drinking it. Soon after that, he began denouncing alcohol in public declarations. What began as a clinical aid and a scientific curiosity ended up as the villainous target of a public campaign.

For many years, Emil Kraepelin believed that drinking was good for you, that it was something people had to do to remain healthy. Doubts developed, however, as he grew older. According to the story he tells in his *Memories*, the turning point came in the spring of 1895 during a vacation in Greece. He was drinking the local specialty, wines fermented with small amounts of pine resin. As he later recalled, "I did not enjoy it at all. As I returned home, I decided that I would finally give up alcohol altogether and fight."[90] Yes, he certainly did fight.

It is impossible to know all the reasons why Kraepelin became an ardent campaigner against alcoholic consumption. His father's alcoholism may have been a factor, but moral considerations were probably more important. Evidence comes, in part, from his own pharmacological experiments. In summarizing those experiments, he wrote that alcohol causes "intellectual stupefaction and moral insanity ... which one is forced to call pathological." And then, this noteworthy qualification, "Of course, there are rather significant individual differences, depending on the primary moral predisposition; insecure souls more easily succumb to the seductive effect of alcohol than strong-minded people."[91] Moreover, when summarizing the entire pharmacopsychology project, he wrote that, "Alcohol, ether, chloroform, chloral hydrate, paraldehyde and morphine produce, if in different strengths, *this persistent weakness of will* ... [italics added].[92]

References to "weakness of will" appear frequently in Kraepelin's writings, as do phrases like "moral insanity" and "strong-minded people". They reflect a moral framework in which strength of will was highly valued. Kraepelin's problem with alcohol was that it weakened the will.

As a university student, Kraepelin "eagerly read" the works of many philosophers (quoted words in his *Memoirs*). Surely in those works, he would have read about the will, or will power, because it was a major subject in German philosophy. In the generation before Kraepelin, Arthur Schopenhauer (1788-1860) wrote at length about will, generally denouncing it as evil and naming it as the source of man's suffering. Kraepelin's contemporary, Friedrich Nietzsche (1844-1900), held to a very different opinion. He took will to be empowering, even going so far as to proclaim will – and the related "will to power" – as the fundamental stuff of nature.

> Granted ... that we succeeded in explaining our entire instinctive life as the development and ramification of one fundamental

---

[90] E. Kraepelin (1987), p. 70.
[91] Steinberg and Angermeyer (2001), p. 309.
[92] U. Müller, P.C. Fletcher and H. Steinberg (2006), p. 133.

form of will – namely, the Will to Power as *my* thesis puts it; granted that all organic functions could be traced back to this Will to Power, and that the solution of the problem of generation and nutrition - it is one problem – could also be found therein: one would thus have acquired the right to define all active force unequivocally as *Will to Power* [italics in original].[93]

In a similar vein, Kraepelin wrote in his *Memoirs* of how his view of life had been affected by travels in southeast Asia.

My general understanding of nature was influenced by the insight into the tropical world. My unclear conception of the basic importance of will in nature became clearer and took on a firm shape. Based on a thousand different phenomena, it became exceptionally clear that in every living being the dormant, impulsive functions of the will control not only his way of life, but also his development and constitution.[94]

Once past university, Kraepelin did not trouble himself with academic philosophy, but he consistently admired strong-willed individuals and loathed the weak-willed. He celebrated every birthday of Otto von Bismarck, the military and political leader who personified authority, power and self-confidence. Contrastingly, he routinely referred to his patients as "weak" and possessed of "failing" wills. In writing about patients diagnosed with *dementia praecox*, for example, he stated,

In the whole conduct of the patients the *devastation of their will* makes itself conspicuous above everything. They are tired, weak, lazy, without initiative, irresolute, let themselves become destitute, live carelessly a day at a time fling away money and possessions senselessly, let themselves drift according to chance influences and therefore come quickly down in the world especially when they begin to drink [italics in original].[95]

Hannah Decker is an historian and authority on Kraepelin's clinical work. After reviewing all his major publications, she wrote that "the stress on the

---

[93]Friedrich Nietzsche, *Beyond Good and Evil,* trans. Helen Zimmern. New York, MacMillan (1886, 1907), section 36, p. 52.

[94]E. Kraepelin (1987), p. 115.

[95]Emil Kraepelin, *Dementia Praecox and Paraphrenia,* trans. Mary Barclay. Edinburgh, E&S Livingstone (1896,1919), pp. 106-107.

will is so omnipresent that the reader cannot help wondering why [he] is so engrossed ... One possible interpretation is that Kraepelin was the last in a long line of philosophers, psychologists, and psychiatrists who, until the end of the nineteenth century, thought of the will as an independent faculty of the mind ...[96]

There can be little doubt that Kraepelin abhorred weak wills. Also, he believed that alcohol either makes wills weak or is itself the consequence weak wills. The coupling of these two attitudes led to his disdain for alcohol. That, plus the conviction that what was bad for the German people must also be bad for the German empire. As a mature man secure in his place, Kraepelin chose to act on behalf of these concerns.

When lecturing to medical students, he told them that alcohol is at the root of many diseases. He stated that alcoholic intoxication on the part of either parent at the time of copulation predisposes the offspring to idiocy. He referred to the striking frequency of alcoholism in the parents of patients diagnosed with *dementia praecox*. Even progressive paralysis – usually attributed to syphilis infection – was linked to alcohol. Alcohol may not be the sole cause of any mental illness, he said, yet there is not a single mental illness that is not worsened by it.

Kraepelin also spoke to secondary school students and the general public. When addressing these lay audiences, he emphasized the fact that alcohol loosens the reins on behavior. It causes us to ignore our moral feelings, and leaves us at the mercy of our primitive impulses. That explains why alcoholics so often commit shameless acts. Finally, he never failed to describe, in gruesome detail, the horrible symptoms of advanced delirium tremens.

Kraepelin's principled stand on abstinence triggered arguments with colleagues and made him the butt of jokes. People stopped inviting him to certain social events on account of his stand. Those slights hardly bothered him because he eschewed such events, but an incident that occurred while on vacation in Italy struck him more deeply. Kraepelin was in a café speaking with some Germans who knew that he was from Heidelberg. In the course of the conversation, his countrymen asked if he had heard about the weird professor who did not drink alcohol. At that point, Kraepelin realized that he had become more famous for his refusal to drink alcohol than he was for his scientific work.

None of this deterred Kraepelin. On the contrary, he converted his personal commitment into an all-out public campaign. He wrote articles for

---

[96]Hannah Decker, "The psychiatric works of Emil Kraepelin: a many-faceted story of modern medicine," *Journal of the History of the Neurosciences* 13:248-276 (2004).

the popular press. He co-founded the Society of Abstinent Physicians. And, most energetically, he organized the Heidelberg branch of the German Society Opposed to the Abuse of Spirituous Liquors. Meeting every week on Saturday evenings, its membership grew from fifty-one to two hundred fifty under Kraepelin's leadership.

Kraepelin suffered from migraine headaches as a young man. He was delighted, therefore, to discover that the headaches stopped when he quit drinking. The broader effects of his advocacy were less clear. No doubt some individuals followed his advice and benefitted from it, but no one noticed any change in the number of students crowding the *Bierstubes* and cafés around Heidelberg.

One day, Kraepelin arrived at the clinic wanting to speak with Nissl. Because it was still early in the morning, Kraepelin went straight to Nissl's apartment, but Nissl was neither there nor in his office. When Kraepelin enquired among Nissl's colleagues, each of them mentioned that Nissl had been drinking beer late into the previous night. They suggested that Kraepelin go down to Nissl's laboratory, and it was there that Kraepelin encountered, lined up outside the laboratory door, a long row of one-liter beer bottles – all empty. Kraepelin was aghast. He took deep breaths. His face flushed red. Just then, Nissl came bounding out the door laughing. "Ha ha," he bellowed, "I fooled you!"

Kraepelin knew Nissl well enough to accept the prank for what it was, a gentle teasing. Clearly, these men had their own personalities and their own, contrasting lifestyles. And yet, despite their differences, Kraepelin and Nissl built a productive relationship based on mutual respect and a common commitment to scientific psychiatry.

13 Psychosis

Seven years after moving to Heidelberg, Kraepelin and his family were still living on *Bergheimer Straße*, in an apartment that was conveniently located but no longer adequate for the growing family, which now included four daughters. His mother also stayed with them from time to time. Fortunately, Emil's earnings from his activities as author, clinic director and consultant had brought him to the point where he could afford larger accommodations.

So, when Kraepelin heard of a grand new house being built on *Scheffelstraße*, on the northern slope of Heiligenberg Mountain, he bought it. The street was named after the poet and novelist Joseph Victor von Scheffel, who had died two years earlier. The house was large enough to easily accommodate the family, its servants and its kitchen personnel. All the rooms had tall ceilings and ornate finishes, and many of them were fitted with telephone connections.

It was the natural setting, however, that Kraepelin liked best. His new home lay immediately in front of a natural forest and adjacent to the gentle landscapes of Philosopher's Walk. The southern facing windows afforded an unobstructed view across the Neckar River to the *Heiliggeistkirche* and, higher up, nestled on the hill above the old town, the haunting castle. To the west lay the Rhine plain, punctuated by the towering cathedral of Speyer, and to the east the green Neckar valley.

In the garden behind the house lay a cozy little cottage, which Kraepelin immediately recognized as a place meant for undisturbed work. Built years earlier as a boys' clubhouse, it was fitted with colonial windows and an attractive gable. Kraepelin hired a local artist to decorate the gable with a flute-playing angel, copied from a painting by the Italian artist, Meloggo da Forli. He installed tables and chairs outside the bungalow so that his family could join him for coffee and cakes.

Sitting comfortably in his garden study, Kraepelin, would have contemplated the puzzle of psychosis. Despite having no precise definition, everyone knew what it was. It was the worst mental affliction, seen only in the maddest of the mad. It was not, however, a single disease, nor even a

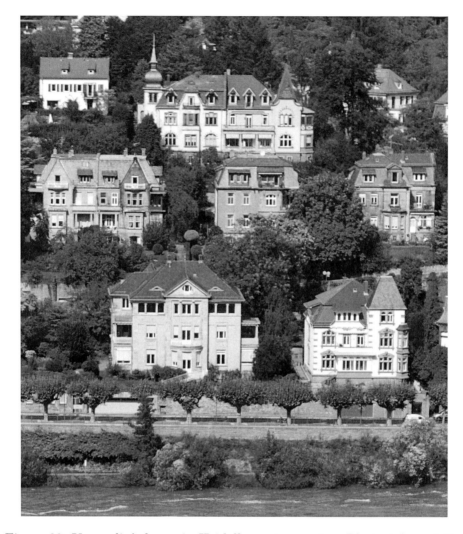

Figure 22: Kraepelin's home in Heidelberg, top center. Photo taken at the Schloss, on the opposite side of the Neckar River (foreground). [R. Chase]

consistent set of symptoms. If a patient seemed to be inhabiting a world of her own, if she described outlandish notions and spoke gibberish, she was likely psychotic. Today we say that patients who lose contact with reality are psychotic. For Kraepelin and his colleagues, psychosis was the most challenging of all mental conditions. They struggled to define it, and they struggled to identify the individual disorders that fell under its rubric.

Most people understand that there is a difference between psychosis and neurosis, but few know the remarkable history of that difference. First came neurosis. Because its definition changed dramatically over time, attention must be paid to the original definition. Originally, a mental condition was a neurosis if it was thought to be caused by a brain abnormality, but there was no actual evidence of any lesion. By that definition, which dates from 1777, even the mental disorders that occasionally accompanied epileptic seizures were known as neuroses. Thus, epileptic insanity was a recognized type of neurosis. Then, in 1845, the Viennese psychiatrist, Ernst von Feuchtersleben, coined the term psychosis. His awkward definition of psychosis, and the distinction that he drew between it and neurosis, caused understandable confusion. He wrote,

> Where psychic phenomena present themselves abnormally, we speak of mental illness; it is rooted in the mind, and insofar as these phenomena are transmitted through the brain, they are rooted in the body because the brain is the organ of the mind... Every psychosis is at the same time a neurosis, because without the mediation of the nervous system no mental change is able to become manifest; but every neurosis is not simultaneously a psychosis.[97]

In other words, every mental illness is rooted in the brain (neurosis), but not every brain problem produces a psychosis. In effect, Feuchtersleben was confirming and expanding the original definition of a neurosis, while introducing psychosis as the term for illnesses that have no basis in brain abnormalities. Somehow, in the ensuing years Feuchtersleben's intended meanings were misread and actually reversed. The result was that neurosis came to mean a *purely psychological disorder*, for example a condition affecting mood, anxiety or conflict, while psychosis meant any type of psychological disorder *caused by a brain disorder*. When it is said that Freud focused on neurotic disorders while Kraepelin focused on psychosis, the distinction is drawn from the revised definitions.

Psychotic disorders (as currently defined) are severely debilitating. They resist treatment, disrupt families and account for high rates of suicide. In the nineteenth century, when psychotic patients were sedated and restrained but otherwise untreated, their bizarre signs and symptoms – involving hallucinations, delusions and nonsensical speech – must have left a

---

[97]Quoted in Edward Shorter, *A Historical Dictionary of Psychiatry*. New York, Oxford University Press (2005), p. 241.

compelling impression on persons attending them. Following Griesinger's call for a scientific psychiatry, and with neuroanatomy developing at a fast pace, many psychiatrists saw psychosis as the most likely of all mental conditions to show signs of brain pathology. The search for evidence occupied Nissl and his fellow psychiatrist-anatomists, but no one found anything of enduring interest. Meanwhile, for clinicians like Kraepelin, who worried about diagnosis and prognosis, psychosis was another sort of problem.

Apart from the psychoses, most cases brought to the attention of a psychiatrist were diagnosed without much difficulty. Epilepsy was recognized by its seizures, loss of memory, impaired judgment and weakmindedness. Progressive paralysis was diagnosed by immobility and dementia, and uniquely in such cases, the diagnosis could be confirmed by postmortem examination of the brain. Alcoholism was more complicated because the signs and symptoms varied with the stage of the disease. Nevertheless, acute alcoholic intoxication was indicated by perceptual and motor dysfunctions of the types observed by Kraepelin in his experimental studies, and chronic alcoholism was indicated by hallucinations, paranoia and delirium tremens. Likewise, obsession, hysteria, imbecility and cretinism, had their distinctive symptoms. Confident though he was in his ability to diagnose the above-named disorders, Kraepelin was much less certain about diagnosing the larger number of cases that fell under the umbrella of psychosis. Although most clinicians had a general idea of what psychosis was, there was no consensus on either its precise definition or the number of separate disorders that belonged to the category.

In the second half of the nineteenth century, psychosis had roughly the same meaning as insanity. In France, it amounted to mania and melancholia, whereas in Germany, it was equivalent to *Wahnsinn*. But confusion reigned. One year after Feuchtersleben introduced the term *Psychose* (1845), another German psychiatrist, Heinrich Damerow, published a textbook in which he listed the terms denoting mental disorder. *Psychosen* (pleural form) is there, but so too are thirteen synonyms,

> *Seelenstörungen, Irresein, Geisteskrankheiten, Verstandesver-*
> *rückungen, Geisteszerrüttungen, Gemüthsstörungen, Gemüths-*
> *krankheiten, Psychosen, Psychoneurosen, Psychopathien, Pre-*
> *nopathien, die sensitiven Krankheiten, Logoneurosen, Persön-*
> *lichkeitskrankheiten, und so weiter* [and so on].[98]

---

[98]Quoted in M. Dominic Beer, "Psychosis: from mental disorder to disease concept," *History of Psychiatry* 6 (1995), p. 156.

The concept of psychosis was in need of repair. Was it just a way of referencing certain severe symptoms, or were there definable psychotic disorders? Some authors still thought of epilepsy and cretinism as psychotic illnesses. Others wanted to include late stage progressive paralysis but not early stage progressive paralysis. So, was it time to cut again at the joints of mental illness or, as some psychiatrists contended, was it time to put the knife away? The latter group of psychiatrists expressed no interest in identifying psychotic disorders. And, they went further, insisting that the entire practice of dissecting mental illness was unnecessary in practice and ill-founded in principle. These men called themselves unitarians, and many psychiatrists, especially in Germany, held to their point of view. The movement advanced under the banner of *Einheitspsychose*, or "unitary psychosis".

The unitarians maintained that there is just a single disease – call it psychosis, insanity, madness or whatever. Trying to carve it up is both senseless and useless. Albert Zeller, the director of an asylum where Wilhelm Griesinger had once apprenticed, wrote that all afflictions of the soul must be united because the soul itself is unified. Other unitarians acknowledged that signs and symptoms differ in different patients but, they claimed, that only indicates different stages in the progression of a single disease. A physician might find that a patient is melancholic. Later, that same patient might progress to paranoia, and eventually to dementia, but it is all just mental illness. Heinrich Neumann, another unitarian theorist put it this way, "Every classification of mental illness is artificial. We should throw it all overboard ... there is only one form of mental illness, that is insanity [*Wahnsinn*], which does not have different forms but different stages."[99] Neumann saw mental illness as a continuum ranging from health to disease. Each degree of sickness has its own characteristic symptoms, but fundamentally, every patient has the same disease.

For psychiatrists tired of fussing over problematic, time-consuming diagnoses, unitary psychosis was an attractive idea. It was welcomed by practitioners who were comfortable dealing in a practical way with individual patients, but puzzled by what they felt were abstract definitions. There was also the fact that the unitarian outlook encouraged early institutionalization, which many psychiatrists saw as beneficial.

The main reason why Kraepelin did not buy into unitarianism, was progressive paralysis. Judging by its name alone, one might imagine that

---
[99]G. E. Berrios and D. Beer, "The notion of unitary psychosis: a conceptual history," *History of Psychiatry* 5 (1994), p. 26.

progressive paralysis offered positive proof of unitary psychosis, for it was a single disease that changed over time. However, while the symptoms were multiple, the illness as a whole was different enough from all other forms of psychosis that no mainstream psychiatrist had any difficulty in accepting progressive paralysis as a distinct illness. In light of this compelling example, Kraepelin decided that unitarianism must be false. That decision, and his recognition of progressive paralysis as a paradigmatic mental illness, later proved pivotal in the construction of his landmark classification.

Described by some as the "disease of the nineteenth century", progressive paralysis was important not just because it killed unitary psychosis, but also because it brought mental illness to the attention of the medical establishment. Its mix of physical and mental symptoms forced doctors to consider each dimension as equal in weight and equally demanding of treatment. There is little record of it prior to 1800, but afterwards it spread like wildfire. It was particularly prevalent among well-educated merchants and military personnel, nearly all of whom were men. By the 1860s, annual statistical reports from a private clinic near Breslau were showing that one-third of the male patients had progressive paralysis, while none of the seventy-five female patients had it. Although many people believed that alcohol was the cause, the true cause turned out to be a bacterium, *Treponema pallidum*. Progressive paralysis is actually a late manifestation of syphilis, which accounts for its later name, neurosyphilis. Overall, millions of people were affected and thousands poured into asylums and clinics. Most of the infected patients died from the illness, including such well-known persons as Friedrich Nietzsche, Franz Schubert and Edouard Manet.

Syphilis had been known since at least the middle ages, but progressive paralysis was not recognized as a disease until 1822. In that year, Antoine Laurent Bayle discovered a physical correlate of the disease in the brains of its victims. Histological methods were not yet good enough to detect cellular pathologies, but Bayle was able to find unmistakable signs of inflammation in the arachnoid membrane, which is a tissue that covers and protects the brain. Many years later, the new breed of anatomically oriented psychiatrists pointed to Bayle's work as an example of biological causation. Franz Nissl's prize-winning stain was initially put to work looking for relevant pathologies. Later, he and Alois Alzheimer collaborated over many years in a study of progressive paralysis, work that began in Frankfurt and continued afterwards in Heidelberg and Munich.

Patients with progressive paralysis typically moved through several stages, usually counted as three or four. Different signs and symptoms characterized each stage. First, there were sores on the penis. Sometimes the sores disappeared and the victims would remain symptom-free for several years, but at some point friends and family members would notice slurred speech and a slight tremor of the lips and tongue. Victims at this stage reported blurred vision, and they complained of not seeing certain colors. Next came the mental symptoms, which were various, running the gamut from mania to dementia. Later still, serious physical problems developed. The patient's gait became ataxic (uncoordinated), the muscles got progressively weaker, and eventually he or she would be unable to move. Seizures followed, and finally death.

The dramatic manic phase produced classic examples of psychotic delusion, many of which were delusions of grandeur. For example, during the reign of Napoleon Bonaparte, more than a few patients believed that *they* were Napoleon. The general nature of the manic phase was described in a medical dictionary published twenty years after Napoleon's death,

> It is above all during this phase that [the patient] totally succumbs to illusions of silly vanity, whether he believes himself to be king, pope, emperor, grandee, millionaire, or owner of vast treasures. This one calls himself Napoleon and has won every battle of empire; another maintains that he has produced all the masterpieces now gracing our museums of painting and sculpture; yet another has only to nod his head to erect magnificent palaces, cities of crystal, houses of diamonds, and he makes bizarre movements; some paralytics think they are thirty feet, or forty or fifty cubits, tall.[100]

Another common theme was profligate spending, as in the case of a chemistry professor in Frankfurt who suddenly went on a spending spree, buying 10 automobiles and 100 wrist watches in a single day.[101] Similar cases were described by Julius Mickle in his classic book on progressive paralysis, originally published in 1880. For example,

> Says his head is bad, will get a new head when he goes to heaven, it was full of diamonds and has been taken off. His

---

[100]Quoted by Laure Murat in *The Man Who Thought He Was Napoleon: Toward a Political History of Madness*. Chicago, University of Chicago Press (2014), p. 113.
[101]E. Shorter (1997), p. 54.

> heart and lungs have been taken out ... Will be a giant 125 feet high, and made so, in sum or heaven, by 7 quarts each of brandy and whisky, and 3 of beer. Has four ducal titles ... is first field-marshal, has millions and millions of gold watches.

The all-to-common consequence of such delusions is noted in this final example from Mickle's book.

> If at large, the delusions lead to the most extravagant projects ... [He] sends telegrams containing preposterous orders, such as to lade a ship with wine, 'for sale in the uninhabited parts of the earth,' and thus, without extraneous aid, these patients often fritter away their means on impracticable or ill-advised business-schemes and speculations.[102]

Writing in the second edition of his treatise (1886), Mickle filled twenty pages with descriptions of pathologies that could be seen with the naked eye, including inflammation of the arachnoid membrane, as reported by Bayle. A further twenty-six pages described microscopic abnormalities, which he divided into three main categories. Within the category blood vessels, he mentions twelve types, within neuroglia (the brain's non-neuronal cells) eleven types, and within nerve cells and fibers, another eleven types. Despite all the current talk about cerebral localization, Mickle found none. He wrote that the pathology characteristic of progressive paralysis was seen everywhere in the cerebral cortex, a result confirmed by Nissl and Alzheimer in their five hundred page review of the disease published in 1904.

Progressive paralysis had everything that a mental disease must have – plenty of signs and symptoms and a grandiose mania that was unquestionably indicative of psychological disturbance. Yes, some signs, like tremors, muscle weakness and paralysis were physical, but by the same token they satisfied the need for a measurable diagnostic criterion. Neural pathology was another objective sign, albeit one that was useless for purposes of diagnosis because it was unavailable until after death. Furthermore, progressive paralysis had a known cause, syphilis infection, and a predictable course from penis sores to dementia and death. Some of Kraepelin's fellow psychiatrists fretted over whether to regard progressive paralysis as fundamentally seated in the mind or in the brain, but he did not. For Kraepelin,

---

[102]Wm. Julius Mickle, *General Paralysis of the Insane*. London, H.K. Lewis (2nd ed., 1886). Quotes on, pp. 42, 45.

it was enough that progressive paralysis was widely accepted as a psychiatric disease. Considering all of its properties, there was no other psychosis quite like it. It was a species of disease as real and unique as a platypus among mammals or a gingko among trees.

Secure now in the knowledge that progressive paralysis was a true illness as well as a type of psychosis, Kraepelin thought to use it as a model for finding additional psychotic illnesses. He vowed to complete some of that work in time for inclusion in the next edition of his textbook, which had already been twice revised. The second and third editions had been prepared in Dorpat, where his attention was divided between experimental psychology and clinical psychiatry. Moreover, due to language difficulties, he had been unable to obtain the kinds of data that he needed for reevaluating the classification. But now, in Heidelberg, he was running his own show. He had ready access to a wide variety of patients, surveillance rooms in which to observe them, and a trusted team of assistants to help him. It was the ideal time to tackle the thorny issue of disease identification.

In the spring of 1893, he took a vacation in Italy. As usual, he mixed pleasure with work. He went first to Parma where he visited a mental asylum in the province of Reggio Emilia. From there, he rode by postal coach through the Apennine Mountains to Santa Margherita, for the purpose of conferring with a professional acquaintance. Finally, he reached the Riviera, hopping from San Remo to Nice, then Cannes and Monte Carlo before heading home. We do not know for sure that he worked on the textbook during this long trip, but he may well have, because by September it was finished.

When the fourth edition of Kraepelin's textbook came out in the fall of 1893, the dedication read, "To the memory of Bernhard von Gudden." Kraepelin introduced a new illness in this book. He called it *dementia praecox* – Latin for precocious dementia – but the name was later changed to schizophrenia. Today, we know schizophrenia as one of the most common and most debilitating of all mental disorders. Delusions and hallucinations are its hallmark symptoms. They cause patients to behave in bizarre ways, drawing attention to themselves and to the illness. Worldwide, about one in every one hundred persons has or will have the illness at some point in their lives. It is, perhaps, the prototypical mental disorder.

Dementia praecox was Kraepelin's prime cut from the body of psychosis. However, Kraepelin did not actually discover *dementia praecox*, as a nautical explorer might discover a small island in the Pacific Ocean or a zoologist might discover a new species of bird. It would be more accurate to say that he *constructed* the disease by reading the psychiatric literature, interviewing patients, and observing patients in surveillance rooms.

As an avid student of the psychiatric and scientific literatures, Kraepelin had surely read case histories from the early years of the nineteenth century that bore the marks of schizophrenia. Phillipe Pinel, for one, had described such cases, but the most striking of all were those written by John Haslam, a Londoner who worked as the apothecary, or pharmacist, at the Bethlem hospital. In his book, *Observations of Madness and Melancholy* (1809), Haslam mentions the case of a young man who "under the supposed imputation of having unnatural propensities" had cut off his penis. The patient also complained "that the boards on which he walked were heated by subterraneous fires, under the direction of invisible and malicious agents, whose intentions, he was well convinced, were to consume him by degrees." At other times, the man was perfectly lucid. According to Haslam, madmen "have sometimes such a high degree of control over their minds, that when they have any particular purpose to carry, they will affect to renounce those opinions, which shall have been judged inconsistent ..."

Elsewhere in the book, Haslam writes about young persons who were disinterested in common activities, lacked social relations and suffered from a loss of memory. "Frequently noticed in females," he wrote, "the disorder commences, about, or shortly after, the period of menstruation, and in many instances has been unconnected with hereditary trait." Mixing genders in the same section, Haslam further stated, "In the interval between puberty and manhood, I have painfully witnessed this hopeless and degrading change, which in a short time has transformed the most promising and vigorous intellect into a slavering and bloated ideot."[103] Notable here are the observations of an illness that develops in young adults, quickly worsens and is manifested by apathy and intellectual deterioration, all of which characterize schizophrenia

These brief case descriptions were but small preludes to the psychosis that Haslam described in his next book, which came with the unwieldy title, *Illustrations of Madness: Exhibiting a Singular Case of Insanity, And a No Less Remarkable Difference in Medical Opinions: Developing the Nature of An Assailment, And the Manner of Working Events; with a Description of*

---

[103] John Haslam, *Observations on Madness and Melancholy*, 2nd edition. London, Callow (1809), pp. 49-51, 64-67.

Tortures Experienced by Bomb-Bursting, Lobster-Cracking and Lengthening the Brain. Embellished with a Curious Plate.

Better known by its shortened title, *Illustrations of Madness*, Haslam's book was published in 1810. The entire book is devoted to the description of a single patient, James Tilley Matthews, who had been brought to the hospital at age twenty-seven and placed under Haslam's care. Matthews was a tea merchant with a wife and children. The French Revolution caused him to worry about a possible war between England and France, so he began traveling back and forth between Paris and London on a self-appointed peace mission. Accused of spying, he spent three years in a French prison. After returning to London, he showed up one day in the public gallery of the House of Commons. There, he stood up and loudly accused the Home Secretary of treason, which explains how he wound up at Bethlem Hospital.

In the Preface to his book – before giving any details regarding Matthews and his insanity – Haslam explains his motivation for writing it.

> The publication of the following case is deemed as much an act of justice, as it may be regarded a matter of curiosity. It may possibly effect some good, by turning the attention of medical men to the subject of professional etiquette ... If it should merely succeed in curbing the fond propensity to form hasty conclusions, or tend to moderate the mischief of privileged opinion, the purpose is sufficiently answered.

It happened that Matthews' family did not believe that he was insane, and they brought a writ of habeas corpus to get him released. Matthews was, indeed, remarkably normal at times, consistent with Haslam's comments in his earlier book. After listening to testimonies from medical and quasi-medical witnesses, the judge stated that Matthews was too dangerous to be released, and he denied the writ. Haslam had been one of the witnesses. Although he agreed with the judge's decision, he was offended by the written judgment because, in his opinion, it gave scant attention to his own testimony. He was so indignant that he wrote *Illustrations of Madness* to correct the judge's omission.

Matthews believed that he was being persecuted by a gang of undercover French revolutionaries who were controlling his mind. He spoke of an elaborate machine, an "air loom" (Figure 23), which the gang used to impose its will upon him. Mike Jay's splendid book tells the full story of James Tilly Matthews.[104] Here is Jay's succinct summary of the air loom,

> [It] combined recent developments in gas chemistry with the strange force of animal magnetism, or mesmerism. It incorporated keys, levers, barrels, batteries, sails, brass retorts and magnetic fluid, and worked by directing and modulating magnetically charged air currents, rather as the stops of an organ modulate its tones. It ran on a mixture of foul substances, including 'spermatic-animal-seminal rays', 'effluvia of dogs' and 'putrid human breath', and its discharges of magnetic fluid were focused to deliver thoughts, feelings and sensations directly into Matthews' brain. There were many of these mind-control settings, all classified by vivid names: 'fluid locking', 'stone making', 'thigh talking', 'lobster-cracking', 'bomb-bursting', and the dreaded 'brain-saying', whereby thoughts were forced into his brain against his will.[105]

Knowing details such as these, one could hardly fault the judge for declaring Matthews insane. He was clearly paranoid, but did he have schizophrenia? According to current criteria, delusions and auditory hallucinations are cardinal symptoms, and Matthews had both. Also indicative are the facts that he became ill at a young age and he apparently did not recover, because he remained in an asylum for the rest of his life. If Matthews were to appear at a clinic today, he would most probably be diagnosed with schizophrenia.

Given Haslam's detailed case study – along with similar, albeit less expansive, accounts written by other early nineteenth century psychiatrists – why was schizophrenia not seen as a distinct mental illness long before Kraepelin identified it many decades later? A modern British psychiatrist, Edward Hare, plunged into old hospital records and government archives in search of an answer. He found, among other things, that prior to 1800, there was not a single, unambiguous record of a patient hearing voices. This striking claim begs an explanation, because auditory hallucinations are highly characteristic of schizophrenia. There are at least two possibilities. First, since lengthy case histories of any kind were uncommon

---

[104]Mike Jay, *A Visionary Madness: The Case of James Tilly Matthews and the Influencing Machine.* Berkeley, CA, North Atlantic Books (2014).

[105]Mike Jay, "The Air Loom Gang: James Tilly Matthews and his visionary madness," http://www.nthposition.com/theairloomgangjames.php.

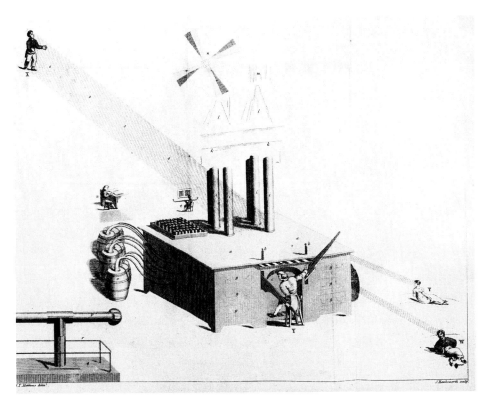

Figure 23: James Tilley Matthews' delusional air loom. Drawn by
Matthews himself, it depicts a gang member operating a machine (center) which transmits thoughts to Matthews (upper
left). [John Haslam, 1810]

until Pinel, Esquirol, Haslam, and a few other alienists starting using them
shortly after the turn of the century, schizophrenia may have gone unno-
ticed in the pared down, simplistic descriptions of earlier times. Insanity
was madness and there was little more to be said about it.

According to a second interpretation, the one favored by Edward Hare,
there were no descriptions of schizophrenia prior to Haslam because there
was no schizophrenia. Recall that asylums were bursting at their seams
in the late nineteenth century, swollen by an influx of new patients. Hare
thinks that at least some of those added numbers were due to patients
suffering from schizophrenia. He claims that "the postulated increase in
the incidence of schizophrenia can account for at least 40% of the increased
prevalence of insanity between 1859 and 1909." Hare speculates that "a

change of a biological kind" occurred around 1800 that made schizophrenia-like disorders more severe and more common.[106] In summary, whether or not schizophrenia existed before 1800 remains an open question.

Although early authors saw cases that seemed to them peculiar and that featured some of the same symptoms present in schizophrenia, no one used any special diagnostic term in referring to those cases. Later however, around the time that Kraepelin was naming and describing *dementia praecox*, other European psychiatrists were also noting a special form of psychosis. Dr. Valentine Magnan, chief psychiatrist at Sainte Anne's Hospital in Paris, was one such psychiatrist.

Magnan was renowned for crafting an elaborate classification of mental illnesses. He was also an outspoken supporter of August Morel's doctrine of degeneration. That Magnan had discovered schizophrenia, or something like it, is illustrated by a story told by Clarence Farrar, an American visitor in Heidelberg. Farrar was on his way back to America when he stopped at Paris, accompanied by Franz Nissl. Once their presence in Paris became known, Nissl was invited to attend one of Magnan's clinical demonstrations. Just prior to Nissl's visit, Magnan had proudly announced the discovery of a new disease, which he named *délire chronique à évolution systématique* [chronic systematized delusional disorder]. Confident that he had found something of great importance, he was anxious to impress his visitor from the famous Heidelberg clinic.

The demonstration took place at Magnan's hospital. Following a few introductory remarks, Magnan proceeded with the actual demonstration, which was nothing more than an interview with a patient who had been diagnosed with *délire chronique à évolution systématique*. Magnan skillfully drew out the man's paranoia and pointed out the many signs of his mental and physical degeneration. Farrar reported what happened next.

> Nissl listened with closest attention, now and then nodding appreciatively as the Frenchman made some fine psychological analysis of symptoms. The presentation complete, Magnan hopefully awaited Nissl's comment. It was brief and to the point: *Ein ganz typicsher Fall von Dementia praecox* [A typical case of *dementia praecox*].[107]

---

[106]Edward Hare, "Schizophrenia as a recent disease," *British Journal of Psychiatry* 153: 521-531 (1988).

[107]C. B. Farrar (1954), p. 623.

According to Farrar, Magnan returned to his office, lowered his head over his desk, and wept. He could not accept that Kraepelin had already described the same disease, and that it was more aptly and more concisely named than his.

$$-//-$$

Kraepelin read the works of many authors while revising his textbook. More than any other, he was most impressed with Karl Kahlbaum. Already in Dorpat, Kraepelin had incorporated several of Kahlbaum's ideas into his inaugural lecture at the university.

Now, it was Kahlbaum, and Kahlbaum's student, Ewald Hecker, who were to provide the case histories that inspired Kraepelin's *dementia praecox*.

Unlike his illustrious contemporaries Gudden and Griesinger, both of whom were professors at prestigious universities, Kahlbaum never held an academic position. His first job was at an asylum in eastern Prussia. Although he had published a major book at the relatively young age of thirty-five, he could not obtain a professorship. Having no better option, he accepted the directorship of a private clinic in Görlitz and later purchased the clinic. With no high platform from which to deliver his insights, his ground breaking ideas were largely ignored until Kraepelin came upon them a quarter century later.

Kahlbaum took his inspiration from Rudolf Virchow, the man credited with identifying many infectious diseases. He insisted that psychiatry would never be accepted as a true medical discipline until it, too, had identified valid diseases. To accomplish that, he advocated using the so-called "clinical method". All aspects of the illness needed to be considered, not just its symptoms. Symptoms, after all, are only the superficial manifestations of illness. Psychiatry needed to discover the true *essence* of its illnesses (again that word).

> The various forms in which mental illness has been known since antiquity, and is still known today, cannot be considered as different species in their own right but only as symptom-clusters which can appear in the course of different disorders. In this regard, they can be compared with the symptom-complexes such as fever, dropsy, jaundice, cachexy [poor health and malnutrition], et cetera, which in earlier times were considered as diseases but which nowadays are considered to be what they truly

are, namely, symptom-clusters capable of being part of different diseases.[108]

It was this concept of disease essence that Kraepelin endorsed and stressed in his Dorpat lecture. Kahlbaum's skepticism regarding neuroanatomy was another theme borrowed by Kraepelin in that lecture. Contrary to the opinion being voiced by Griesinger, Kahlbaum was less than optimistic about neuroanatomy's potential for delivering useful information. "How wrong it inevitably was to expect pathological anatomy alone to reform the obsolete psychiatric framework."[109] Kraepelin was of like mind, at least initially. Commenting in his *Memoirs* on his attempt to use brain sections for diagnostic purposes – back in 1879 – he recalled, "We were not even capable of differentiating between the cerebral cortex from a paralytic [patient with progressive paralysis of the insane] and from a healthy person, let alone recognizing a certain disease process from the anatomic appearance."[110]

Far more informative, according to Kahlbaum, were the temporal aspects of the illness. This was the single most useful idea that Kraepelin got from Kahlbaum. Psychiatrists tended to assess patients when they were first admitted to the asylum, but rarely afterwards. Therefore, when trying to sort out the various types of disorder, a psychiatrist would typically review the signs and symptoms of his patients, all of whom had been assessed at the time of admission. Alternatively, a psychiatrist might interview all previously admitted patients during a single period of investigation. The technical term for both methodologies is "cross-sectional", meaning that they cut through the patient population at a single moment in time.

In contrast to the cross-sectional methods, Kahlbaum advocated a "longitudinal" approach, whereby the entire course of a patient's illness was to be considered, from onset to final outcome. Acute versus chronic conditions had to be distinguished, as well as changing symptoms over time. Furthermore, he felt it important to note the patient's age at the onset of his or her illness, because normal developmental events can affect disease processes. Kahlbaum believed that all these temporal elements – when considered alongside symptoms and causes – would provide a solid basis for identifying and classifying mental diseases.

---

[108]Karl Kahlbaum, "The clinico-diagnostic perspective in psychopathology," translated by G.E. Berrios. *History of Psychiatry* 18:233-245 (1878, 2007), quote on p. 237.

[109]Karl Kahlbaum, *Catatonia*, translated by Y. Levij and T. Pridan. Baltimore, Johns Hopkins University Press (1874, 1973), p. 2.

[110]E. Kraepelin (1987), p. 16.

In 1863, Kahlbaum published a hefty book with the strangely redundant title, *Die Gruppirung der Psychischen Krankheiten und die Eintheilung der Seelenstörungen* (*The Classification of Mental Diseases and the Division of Psychic Disturbances*). It contained the concrete results of his essence-driven approach to disease identification. He began by discussing more than forty historical classifications from various authors. Next came his own classification, which was complex. Modelled after the biological classifications of Carl Linnaeus, it comprised a hierarchical structure of mostly Latin terms. The following simplified summary is taken from an English language book review of Kahlbaum's *Die Gruppirung*. The review is credited to "H.M.", presumably Henry Maudsley, the renowned British psychiatrist.[111] Note the reliance on temporal factors.

Class I. Neophrenia. Deficiency of mind, produced before, at, or after birth in the first years of life. Including,

- Genera *Innata, Morbosa, Careus*

Class II. Paraphrenia. Mental derangement arising in connection with a transition period of development. Including,

- Genus *Bebetica,* appearing at the time of puberty.

Class III. Vecordia. Idiopathic [of unknown cause] derangement of limited extent as regards mental symptoms (monomania), mostly appearing after puberty. Including,

- Family Dysthymia. Disturbance of feeling or disposition.

- Family Paranoia. Including,

  - Genera *Ascensa, Descensa, Immota*

- Family Diastrephia. Disturbance of the will.

- Family Insania. Without any particular direction of disturbance.

  - Genera *Religiosa, Ethica*

---

[111]H. M., Review of *Die Gruppirung der Psychischen Krankheiten und die Eintheilung der Seelenstörungen, British Journal of Psychiatry* 9:231-233 (1863).

Class IV. Vesania. Idiopathic [of unknown cause] derangement of a general character, affecting all or nearly all mental activity. Including,

- Genus *Typica*, including,
  - Species *T. completa* (four stages), *T. simplex, T. praeceps.*
- Genus *Progressiva,* including,
  - Species *P. complex, P. divergens, P. apoplectica*

Class V. Dysphrenia. Derangement in connection with a physiological or pathological condition of the body. Including,

- Families Nervosa, Chymosa, Sexualis

At the close of his review, Maudsley wrote, "To the author's ingenuity, industry, and learning, his classification is certainly an excellent testimony; but we fear that it is much too theoretical, and that it will not be applicable in practice." Most psychiatrists across Europe were of the same opinion.

Buried and nearly forgotten in *Die Gruppirung*, Kahlbaum briefly mentions *hebephrenia*, one of his many neologisms, but he includes no description. A few years later, Kahlbaum's student, Ewald Hecker, did publish case histories, and it was these descriptions of *hebephrenia* that led Kraepelin to his concept of *dementia praecox.* Details of Kraepelin's journey from *hebephrenia* to *dementia praecox* will be given below, after first noting another of Kahlbaum's enduring contributions.

A few years after *Die Gruppirung*, Kahlbaum started lecturing about what he thought was yet another mental illness. He called it catatonia. Physicians had long recognized a variety of movement disorders. Some physicians saw them as neurological problems, others saw them as psychological problems, and the rest were unsure. If a woman does not move, is it because she *cannot* move or because she *will* not move? Should she be referred to a neurologist or a psychiatrist? Prior to the nineteenth century, it really did not matter, because neurology and psychiatry were effectively blended as a single specialty. Nevertheless, different labels were attached to different types of movement disorders.

The victims of catalepsy, for example, experienced a sudden, transient paralysis accompanied by a total indifference to sensory stimuli. After recovery, the person would remember nothing of the event. Hysteria was another predecessor of catatonia. Although the term later took on other meanings, hysteria was initially associated with abnormal body movements.

Thomas Willis, the Renaissance doctor who had a passion for autopsies and who coined the term neurologie, described the symptoms of hysteria in ample detail,

> ... a choking in the throat, a vertigo, an inversion, or rolling about of the eyes, often-times laughing, or weeping, absurd talking, sometimes want of speech, and motionless, with an obscure or no pulse, and deadish aspect, sometimes convulsive motions, in the face and limbs, and sometimes in the whole body, are excited: but universal convulsions rarely happen ... I have observed these symptoms in maids before ripe age, also in old women after their flowers have left them; yea, sometimes the same kinde of Passions infest men.[112]

In addition to catalepsy and hysteria, there was also *melancholia attonita*. Patients with this disorder were highly depressed, often falling into a kind of stupor and refusing to eat. In 1873, one year before Kahlbaum described catatonia, Dr. S. W. D. Williams, superintendent of the Sussex Lunatic Asylum, reported a partial cure for *melancholia attonita* by means of electrical stimulation. He used, "a continuous current through [the] head from a 40-cell Stohrer's battery [voltage unknown]." He modestly proclaimed,

> to have been greatly impressed with the rapid and satisfactory manner in which these two cases began to recover immediately the electric current was passed through their brains, as though the functions of the great nervous centres were suddenly, by the action of the current, caused to act, and the stupor in which the patients lay previously was dissipated almost before one's eyes.[113]

Kahlbaum gathered together all these disorders – *melancholia attonita*, catalepsy and hysteria – into the single illness, catatonia. In his large book devoted entirely to this one disorder, he defined it this way,

> Catatonia is a brain illness with a cyclic, changing course, in which the psychic symptoms are in turn melancholia, mania,

---

[112]Thomas Willis, *An Essay on the Pathology of the Brain and Nervous Stock*. London, Dring, Harper and Leigh (1681), pp. 76-78.

[113]S. W. D. Williams, "On the treatment of *melancholia attonita*, with refusal of food, by the continuous current," *The Lancet* 101: 127-128 (1873).

stupor, confusion and finally dementia. One or more of these symptoms may be absent from the complete series of psychic 'symptom-complexes'. Besides these psychic symptoms, loco-motor neural processes with the general character of muscular tension occur as typical symptoms.[114]

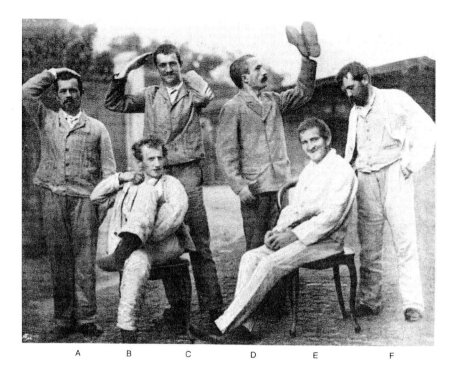

A   B   C   D   E   F

Figure 24: Catatonic patients in Heidelberg. "The patients were easily got into the unusual positions and maintained them as they were photographed in a group, some with roguish smiles, others with rigid solemnity. Of these patients, only E was already quite demented, while A, B and C in particular, were still in the beginning of the disease." [Kraepelin, 1899, v. II, p. 125]

Fifteen years after the publication of Kahlbaum's *Catatonia*, Kraepelin was working in Dorpat, stuck in a place that he did not like and where he was unable to speak the language of his patients. Recalling that time in his *Memoirs,* he wrote,

---

[114]K. Kahlbaum (1874, 1973), p. 83.

I was interested in the question of catatonia and tried to determine whether catatonic symptoms, in particular the command automatism, were characteristic for a certain disease. I was gradually forced to consider the importance of the course of the illness with regard to the classification of the mental disorder. However, I did not come to any clear conclusions, because I had no opportunity to survey the entire development of the disorder from the beginning until the final result in a larger number of patients.[115]

Kraepelin did get an opportunity to "survey the entire development" of catatonia, in Heidelberg, and it was from these longitudinal observations – along with others for related disorders – that he crystallized his notion of *dementia praecox*.

---

[115]E. Kraepelin (1987), pp. 43-44.

14 *Dementia praecox*

When Karl Kahlbaum moved to Görlitz, he brought his student with him and made him his assistant physician. There was a chemistry between Kahlbaum and Ewald Hecker that proved to be productive in the hunt for new mental illnesses. It was, in a way, the chemistry of opposites,

> Isolated and without encouragement or opportunity to exchange ideas, Kahlbaum was beginning to withdraw into his own world. In the young Hecker he found a keen pupil who took up his views with the other perfectly: on the one hand, there was the austere, stern, reserved, organized scientist; on the other an amazingly flexible and warm-hearted pupil, thirsty for new ideas.[116]

Even before moving to Görlitz, Kahlbaum had already "found" *hebephrenia*. He regarded it as a type of paraphrenia, meaning a mental illness that occurs at a particular stage of human development, in this case puberty. The name comes from Hebe, the Greek goddess of youth. Since Kahlbaum gave only a minimal description of *hebephrenia* in his *Die Gruppirung* book, Hecker started taking notes on those of his patients whom he thought represented typical cases. The result was a small article published in the journal, *Archiv für pathologische Anatomie und Physiologie und für klinische Medizin* (Archive for Pathological Anatomy and Physiology and Clinical Medicine). The title of the article (in translation) could not have been more simple or more modest, "Hebephrenia. A contribution to clinical psychiatry."[117]

Hecker's article contains detailed descriptions of seven cases – five males and two females. All patients were between the ages of seventeen and twenty-three years at the time of their first symptoms. Hecker considered case number one a model case. When this patient, Theodor K, arrived at the asylum,

---

[116]Karl Wilmanns, "Eward Hecker (1843-1909)," translated by A. Kraam and G.E. Berrios. Classic Text No. 52, *History of Psychiatry* 13: 458-465 (1924, 2002), quote on pp. 458-459.

[117]Edward Hecker, "Hebephrenia. A contribution to clinical psychiatry," translated by A. Kraam. Classic text no. 77, *History of Psychiatry* 20: 87-106 (1871, 2009).

[He stood] five foot one inch tall, thin, quite malnourished. Head without deformities, face pale, expressionless, and silly. Big eyes, light blue, staring (both pupils equal in size) at the questioner with a blank expression or casting them over the ceiling back and forth. The patient gives correct information about his personality and his background, but keeps inserting into his speech silly remarks, screams suddenly without motive, knocks with his feet on the floor and swerves with his arms and hands clumsily, just like young people in the so-called 'naughty years'. He talks a lot to himself and does not take part in activities or conversation. Instead he does all sorts of silly things: Looking into the bright sun for a long time, hopping on one leg, running back and forth aimlessly, spinning in one spot with eyes closed and head bent backwards in a quick whirl, rubbing his eyes with grass and answering all questions addressed at him with the words: 'But the eyes'.

Hecker included excerpts from his patients' letters, claiming that they were "crucial for the completion of the clinical picture." The following excerpt is from a letter that Theodor K. sent to his parents. Hecker states that the author was using "a Jewish jargon".

And when it evening became our apples and pears they all gone were but instead of the mush we had we had beer soup and when the beer soup was all gone there a small minute 60 passed then before our house there was set alight a big firework ... and today following that I would like to enquire how the German farmers and foresters spend their time there whether they kill it. Yes what is written XXIV that is X and X and again a 4 that is the 24th agricultural and forestry meeting in K. But there has not been one before. The 24th meeting of German farmers and foresters are they walking around naked a lot or what are they doing.

Kraepelin read Hecker's article and was impressed by its wealth of detail, but not totally convinced that hebephrenia was a real disease. He needed firsthand confirmation, and fortunately, he was able to get it from his own student and assistant physician, Leon Daraszkiewicz. Just as Hecker had taken notes on his hebephrenia patients, so too had Daraszkiewicz described more than twenty cases for *his* doctoral dissertation. Again, Kraepelin was impressed with the clinical detail and the intelligent interpretations. Moreover, he was reassured by the fact that Daraszkiewicz's descriptions closely resembled Hecker's. The only difference was that Daraszkiewicz's cases seemed more severe.

In discussions, Daraszkiewicz convinced Kraepelin that many of their demented patients (seen in cross-section) were actually in the late stages of a hebephrenic illness, not imbeciles with an inherited mental deficiency, as many people supposed. He supported the argument by pointing to cases in which patients were simultaneously demented and psychotic. He did not believe that these patients were imbeciles, because in most cases the mental deterioration appeared after, not before, the psychosis. Kraepelin understood the significance of these observations. Hebephrenia, he concluded had a characteristic progression over time. Needing no further proof that hebephrenia was a real disease, Kraepelin decided to include it in the fourth edition of his textbook, albeit under a new name, *dementia praecox*.

Over time, Kraepelin collected a vast store of clinical observations from his and his students' firsthand experiences. Consequently, in writing about *dementia praecox* in every edition of his textbook from the fourth through the ninth, he was able to elucidate the illness by means of lengthy descriptions. In the eighth edition (1913), the last before his death, he mentions no less than thirty-six psychological symptoms, among which hallucinations, catatonic excitement, delusions, memory loss, and the "weakening of volitional impulses".[118] In addition, he mentions nineteen bodily symptoms, including the following.

> The tendon reflexes are generally heightened, often very greatly; in many cases there is also increased mechanical excitability of the muscles and nerves. The pupils are frequently strikingly dilated, particularly in the states of excitement; now and then, distinct but changing pupillary difference is observed, and also restlessness of the eyeball. Also common are vasomotor disturbances, cyanosis, localized edema and dermographia in all gradations; in certain cases there is strong perspiration. Salivation appears to be increased in many cases ... Cardiac activity is subject to great variations, now slowed down, more often slightly accelerated, often also weak and irregular. The body

---

[118]E. Kraepelin, *Dementia Praecox and Paraphrenia*, translated by R. Mary Barclay. Bristol, England, Thoemmes Press (1913, 2002), pp. 5-73. The original work formed part of Kraepelin's textbook on psychiatry, eighth edition.

temperature is mostly low; I once saw it go down to 33.8 C. Menstruation tends to cease or become irregular.[119]

Imitating Hecker, perhaps, Kraepelin also provided paragraph after paragraph of characteristic behaviors and utterances, such as this,

> In the sky there appears a white star, pictures of saints, Christ on the cross ... color pictures are shown on the wall; angels, devils, ghosts, wild animals, snakes and the hell bound appear in the room; flames flare up; human heads are in the food, worms in the soup. Outside, cocks crow, chains rattle, music plays, children wail. God speaks to the patient; the devil calls his name; the whole course of his life is recounted to him. People know his thoughts, talk about him, speak of 'murder and such stories' ... There are revelations, spiritual voices, 'vocal interventions', ventriloquists; when the patient thinks something, he immediately hears it being related to others. In the room there is a vapor, mephitic air, a smell of death; the meal there is human flesh and garbage. Electric currents circulate in his body; other people's blood is pumped in the patient's head and his penis made stiff; the bed makes gestures; 'large frogs crawl into the mouth through the nose and ear.'[120]

And again like Hecker, Kraepelin supplemented his own commentaries with texts written by the patients themselves. Below, is an extract from a lengthy statement written by a female musician five weeks after the onset of her illness.

> In the following night I was electrified. I conclude that from the fact that the following morning I felt quite peculiar pains and twitchings, and it was called out to me a few days before by an electrical machine, which had inspired me with all possible moods and thought, and by mean of which each thought is understood ... Since that day I have had terrible stories of murder and theft in my head, which, as I know that the machine is still always working on me, can absolutely not be controlled ...

---

[119]Emil Kraepelin, *Psychiatry: A Textbook for Students and Physicians*, edition 6, vol. 2, edited by J. Quen, translated by S. Ayed. Cambridge, MA, Science History Publications (1899, 1990), p. 110.

[120]E. Kraepelin (1899, 1990), pp. 120-121.

> horrible smells from time to time, I don't know how, are trans-
> mitted to me. When the physician examined me such plague
> smells also streamed out, that the doctor went backwards ter-
> rified... One evening it was called out to me by the machine:
> 'We conjecture in you the murderer of the Empress of Austria
> (!!!).'[121]

A reader may recognize resemblances between Kraepelin's case descriptions and John Haslam's account of James Tilley Matthews. The percep-
tive reader may also notice that many of the signs and symptoms evident in
the preceding quotations are not unique to *dementia praecox*. They could
equally well have been found in a description of melancholia, mania, or
delirium. However, it was not the signs and symptoms that constituted the
sought-after essence of *dementia praecox*. Rather it was the combination of
early onset, rapid deterioration, and ultimate dementia that uniquely defined the illness. Together, these properties satisfied Kahlbaum's definition
of essence.

Kraepelin's decision to name the illness *dementia praecox* served to distinguish two types of dementia, one occurring in young people (*dementia
praecox*), the other in old people (senile dementia). Senile dementia was
considered irreversible, and Kraepelin initially believed that the dementia
of *dementia praecox* was also irreversible, but he later changed his mind,
agreeing that remissions in *dementia praecox* were sometimes possible.

Kraepelin's choice of the name *dementia praecox* may have been apt,
but it was hardly original. The fact that similar names had been used by
other authors is a good indication that they, too, were familiar with the
disease. Although none of these psychiatrists wrote extensively about it,
their choice of terms indicates that they recognized precocious onset as the
key feature. Heinrich Schüle, working at an asylum in Baden, had referred
to *das pubische Irresein* (pubic insanity); the Parisian psychiatrist, Albert
Charpentier, had written about *les démences de la puberté* (dementias of
puberty); and Benedict Morel had used the term *démence précoce* (precocious dementia). Also, Thomas Clouston, in Edinburgh, had described
what he called "adolescent insanity and its secondary dementia". And
lastly, Arnold Pick, a German professor teaching at Charles University in
Prague, had referred to the hebephrenia of Kahlbaum and Hecker as the
soon-to-be familiar, *dementia praecox*.

---

[121]E. Kraepelin (1913, 2002), p. 110.

Despite Kraepelin's conviction that he had come upon a real mental illness, there were no truly essential features other than the temporal aspects. He would have dearly liked pathological markers, as in progressive paralysis, but there were none. Hecker had been similarly disappointed. He wrote in his article that an anatomist colleague had examined the brain of case number five – postmortem, of course – but found nothing abnormal. Hecker carefully remarked, "The ultimate evidence that hebephrenia stands as a unitary mental illness in its own right can only be provided by pathologic-anatomic facts. But considering the uncertainty provisionally associated with the pathological anatomy of the brain we probably have to dispense with this proof for a long time."

Moreover, again unlike progressive paralysis, there was no probable cause. Hecker was no more troubled by this fact than he was by the absence of neuropathology. "The conclusion that there is a common single cause for such a unified complex of symptoms with a specified and exactly predictable course is not entirely correct but frequently also applied in other fields without objection. The formation of disease entities like cholera, typhoid, Morbus Basedowii [Graves' Disease], et cetera, demonstrates this."

Although Kraepelin could not pinpoint any single cause of *dementia praecox*, he had plenty of ideas. According to degeneration theory, degenerate families carried hereditary defects. From this, Kraepelin considered the possibility that a disruption of normal brain development could cause *dementia praecox*. However, that scenario predicted a slowly developing disorder, whereas *dementia praecox* appeared suddenly and worsened rapidly. Kraepelin ultimately rejected the idea of developmental defects, but ironically, faulty brain development is now seen as the most likely precursor of schizophrenia. Kraepelin also considered Darwinian theory, which suggested that early events in the "struggle for survival" might trigger premature dementia. Kraepelin found that certain of his clinical cases did indeed have difficult childhoods, but not always. Lacking any proof one way or the other with respect to these ideas, he settled on the notion of multiple causation, citing both heredity *and* the environment – which is more-or-less the current view.

In addition to the putative causes mentioned above, Kraepelin also believed that a toxin must, somehow, be involved. Like Nissl in his rabbit experiments, Kraepelin assumed that even common drugs were toxic and thus capable of causing mental illness. He had witnessed the adverse effects of drugs in his experimental studies, and he knew from personal experience the destabilizing effects of alcohol, morphine and possibly cannabis. Mostly, however, he drew upon the example of myxedema, the psychotic disorder caused by lack of thyroid hormone. Kraepelin strongly suspected that a toxin was responsible for damaging the thyroid gland. In light of the fact that *dementia praecox* begins at puberty, Kraepelin thought that it might be caused by a toxic substance affecting the sexual organs.

Just as the cause of *dementia praecox* was unknown, so too was its treatment. A few physicians had recommended castration as a treatment for psychosis, but Kraepelin's speculations notwithstanding, he could not bring himself to try it. However, he did try injecting patients with extracts of testes. When those trials proved ineffective, he gave up on the sexual speculation. He noticed that his patients seemed more normal when feverish, so he thought of raising their body temperature. Cognizant of the association between fevers and high levels of white blood cells, he tried to increase the production of white blood cells by injecting patients with sodium nucleinate, a compound related to DNA. Unfortunately, none of the patients so treated showed any sign of improvement. In the end, Kraepelin fell back on bed rests and baths, and sedation when necessary. As a bit of practical advice for psychiatrists and nurses, he recommended providing patients with good nutrition, sufficient sleep and a bit of exercise.

Finally, Kraepelin considered how to prevent *dementia praecox*, "especially if the malady had been already observed in the parents or brothers and sisters." He thought it best to avoid the dangerous influences "of effeminacy, of poverty, and of exact routine, and especially of city education." He recommended a "childhood spent in the country with plenty of open air, bodily exercise, education beginning late without ambitious aims, and simple food."[122] Such was the state of psychiatric prevention and treatment as late as 1913.

$$-//-$$

Once the dust had settled – from questions about priority and terminology – it was Kraepelin and *his* disease, *dementia praecox*, that came out in front. It was a triumph of sorts, although it was not celebrated. His patients were unaware of the discovery and, since the disease was untreatable, little changed in their lives – with one exception. Kraepelin was struggling to maintain control of admissions and discharges at his clinic, fighting off government bureaucrats who had their own priorities. He was convinced

---

[122]E. Kraepelin (1913, 2002), p. 279.

that dementia was inevitably downhill and irreversible. So, even for a patient diagnosed in the early stages of *dementia praecox*, there was no point in keeping him or her in a clinic dedicated to training and research. Since the subsequent course of the illness was predictable and unavoidable, nothing more could be learned from that patient. Better, to send her to a rural asylum for custodial care and free up the bed for a new, perhaps more interesting, patient. More patients were in fact moved, probably worsening their lives, but providing better opportunities for Kraepelin and co-workers.

Always the patriot, Kraepelin saw that his discovery could also benefit the German military. He was aware of stories in which cowardly men had feigned imbecility in order to avoid military service. Usually an officer would investigate. If he found that the man had seemed normal before his induction – according to testimonies from family and friends – he would conclude that the soldier was simulating, and he would punish him. Kraepelin knew that *dementia praecox*, in its stages, could sometimes masquerade as imbecility. Moreover, he knew a few *dementia praecox* patients who had fluent speech prior to their mental collapse. Some had achieved academic success or performed well in demanding jobs. He, therefore, informed military authorities that they should investigate further before punishing dull, uncooperative soldiers who were found to have acted normally in earlier years.

In 1896, or perhaps slightly before then, Kraepelin began using *dementia praecox* as a diagnostic term. Figure 25 shows a portion of the patient list at the Heidelberg clinic for the year 1900. Six cases are listed as "*dem. praecox*", with ages between sixteen and thirty-two years at the time of admission. Other diagnoses include "Katatonie," "Paralyse," and "Paranoia".

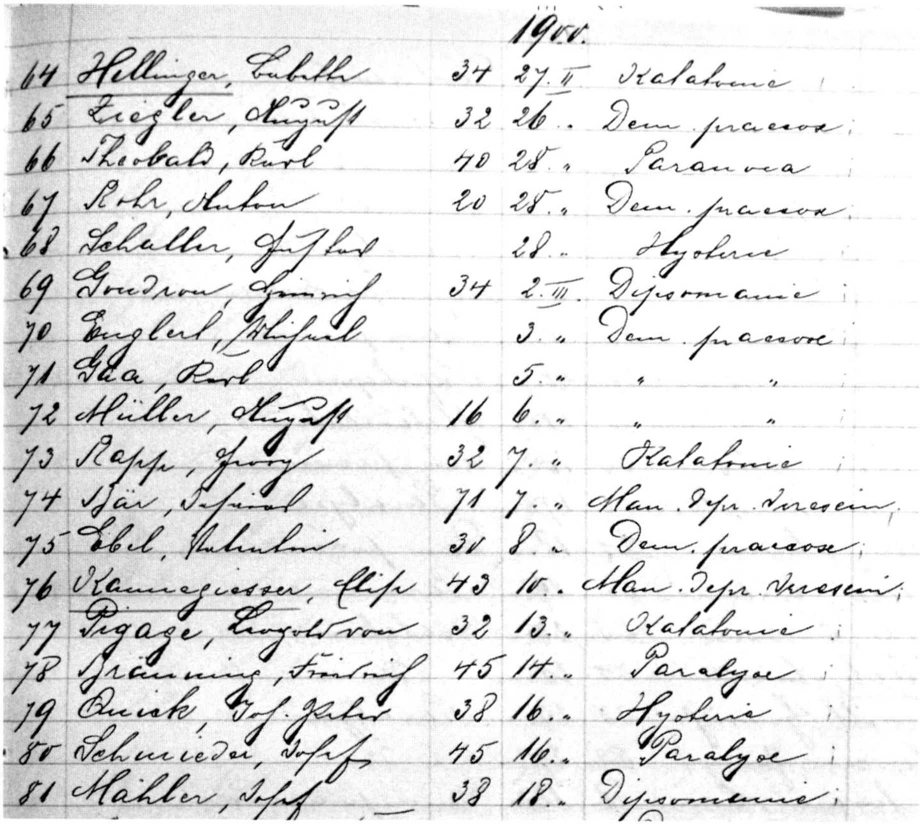

			1900.	
64	Hellinger, Babette	34	27. II	Katatonie
65	Ziegler, August	32	26. "	Dem. praecox
66	Theobald, Karl	40	28. "	Paranoia
67	Rohr, Anton	20	25. "	Dem. praecox
68	Schaller, Gustav		28. "	Hysterie
69	Goudron, Heinrich	34	2. III.	Dipsomanie
70	Englert, Michael		3. "	Dem. praecox
71	Gaa, Karl		5. "	" "
72	Müller, August	16	6. "	" "
73	Rapp, Georg	32	7. "	Katatonie
74	Bär, Daniel	71	7. "	Man. depr. Irresein
75	Ebel, Valentin	31	8. "	Dem. praecox
76	Kammgiesser, Elise	43	10. "	Man. depr. Irresein
77	Pigage, Leopold von	32	13. "	Katatonie
78	Bräunning, Friedrich	45	14. "	Paralyse
79	Quick, Jos. Xaver	38	16. "	Hysterie
80	Schneider, Josef	45	16. "	Paralyse
81	Mähler, Josef	38	18. "	Dipsomanie

Figure 25: Patient list at the Heidelberg psychiatric clinic, 1900. [R. Chase]

15 A Classification for the Twentieth Century

One gets the impression that Kraepelin was constantly at work, whether seeing patients in the clinic, administering, supervising experiments or preparing manuscripts.

Undoubtedly, he was a serious person who worked with a prodigious energy, but he found a balance in life. He had a family, and he also enjoyed the company of a small group of close colleagues. Although he had cordial relations with other professors, he avoided banquets and formal events as much as possible. He preferred hanging out with his male friends, outdoors and actively.

He once led eight co-workers on an excursion down the Neckar River to the picturesque village of Neckarsteinach. A photograph of the group shows the psychiatrists wearing woolen jackets, starched white shirts and black ties – all except Nissl, who hated ties. On a high slope overlooking the river valley lay the ruins of a twelfth century castle. It was there, no doubt, that the group stopped to enjoy their picnic lunch and discuss ... one can only imagine.

For personal fitness, he bought a bicycle and took long trips. Once, while visiting in Munich with Ina, he set out by himself for Lake Constance to consult with a colleague. From there, he cycled to Stuttgart and then to Ernstthal, covering more than five hundred kilometers in just a few days. Pedaling bikes in those days over distances along unpaved or poorly paved roads, as Kraepelin did, was no small feat.

By his own account, Kraepelin spent at least one or two months every year away from Heidelberg. When traveling in Europe, he mixed business and pleasure, whereas in the Canary Islands, North Africa and Southeast Asia it was almost entirely tourism. He had a special fondness for Italy. Once he was able to afford it (near the end of his stay in Heidelberg), he bought a lovely vacation villa in the hilly Piedmont region. In London, he attended the theatre, but found the productions less good than those back home in Germany. As for the five-month trip with his brother to Ceylon

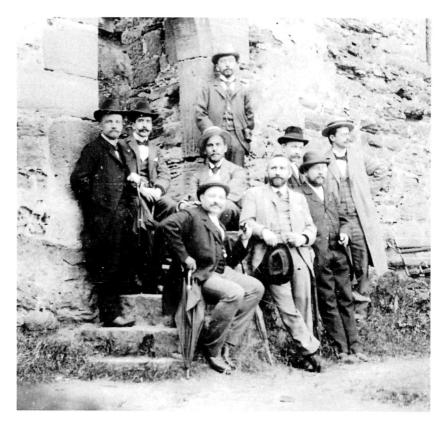

Figure 26: Excursion to Neckarsteinach, 1898. Nissl (left), Kraepelin (right) in front row. [Archive Max-Planck Institute of Psychiatry MPIP-K16/C]

(now Sri Lanka), South India, Singapore and Java, he said of it, "I never felt so happy my entire life as I did on this journey."

At home in Heidelberg, Kraepelin relaxed while walking on the nearby Philosopher's Walk. For more strenuous exercise, he hiked along hilly ridges and explored silent, wooded valleys. As he hiked, he would have been alert to the various plants and animals that he encountered along the way. And, thanks to his brother Karl's instruction during their youthful walks in Neustrelitz, he would have known the names and unique features of each species. It must have crossed his mind that he now possessed a related kind of knowledge, one gained from observing and interviewing patients. Could he use this knowledge to cut further into the body of mental illness, to find all the joints both large and small?

Kraepelin is remembered today mostly for two things: his description of *dementia praecox* (schizophrenia) and his classification of mental illnesses. Neither, however, was achieved at a single point in time. Rather, throughout his career he fiddled with both the definition of *dementia praecox* and the specification of illness groupings in his classification. All of that was made difficult by the fact that everything in psychiatry was in flux: symptom descriptions, psychological versus biological interpretations, disease definitions, disease names and causes.

To keep up with the latest developments, Kraepelin read books and medical journals, but there was nothing like person-to-person discussions. It was one of the reasons that he traveled so often, to learn from his colleagues and listen to their ideas. In the end, though, it was his responsibility to sort through all the information, size it up against his own experience, and arrive at defensible conclusions. Moreover, it was sometimes necessary to change one's mind. Kraepelin's maneuvering with respect to *dementia praecox*, alone, leads us to believe that he gave considerable attention to revising his classification.

Dementia praecox first appeared in the fourth edition of Kraepelin's textbook (1893). The table of contents for that book shows *dementia praecox* placed, along with Kahlbaum's catatonia and *dementia paranoides*, in the category of Degenerating Psychological Processes. It was one of thirteen major categories, each with its own sub-entries. The major categories included old standards such as delirium, mania, melancholia, *dementia paralytica* (progressive paralysis), plus a few new ones, including chronic intoxication and acute exhaustion. Also included were the traditional German terms, *Wahnsinn*, for insanity, and *Verrücktheit*, translating as "craziness" but associated with paranoid delusions.

Psychiatrists were well acquainted with delusions, whether of the paranoid variety or not, yet they puzzled over their place in respect to diagnosis. Were delusions the defining feature of one particular disease, perhaps delirium, or were they merely a symptom common to many different diseases? And, was there a fundamental difference between "ordinary" delusions and paranoid delusions? Opinions varied. Jean-Etienne Esquirol saw delusions as obsessional, hence symptomatic of monomania. Wilhelm Griesinger claimed that delusions rarely occur in the midst of a full-blown insanity, but only *afterwards* as a "secondary state" or a "partial insanity".

By Kraepelin's time, it was widely assumed that delusions were just a symptom of undifferentiated psychosis. Kraepelin broke from that convention by introducing *dementia paranoides* in the fourth edition of his textbook. It was a disorder uniquely characterized by paranoid delusions. He saw it as related to, but distinct from, *dementia praecox*. Whereas as delusions were either absent or of minor importance in *dementia praecox*, they were dominant in *dementia paranoides*. *Verrücktheit* also involved delusions, but somewhat differently. In Kraepelin's conception, *Verrücktheit* was a "durable delusional system in the presence of an intact personality." Unlike patients ill with *dementia paranoides* who were delusional *and* demented, those with *Verrücktheit* were delusional but not totally deteriorated.

Kraepelin placed *dementia praecox* alongside catatonia and *dementia paranoides* in a single category, because all three disorders worsened with time and ended in dementia. His use of the word "degenerating" in the category title, Degenerating Psychological Processes, was descriptive, because degeneration implies progressive deterioration. But "degenerating" also hinted to the then-popular theory of degeneration. Kraepelin himself was skeptical of that theory, but he may have thought it diplomatic to at least allude to the theory in this context. Rather than giving any detailed account of the degenerative processes said to characterize *dementia praecox*, *dementia paranoides* and catatonia, Kraepelin instead substituted metaphors such as "melting" and "dissolving".

Foretelling future sub-typing exercises, Kraepelin mentioned two "forms" of *dementia praecox* in this first description of the illness. He distinguished a milder type, as described by Ewald Hecker, and a more severe type as described by Leon Daraszkiewicz.

Kraepelin tweaked many details of the classification in the next edition of his textbook, the fifth. Briefly, *dementia praecox* (with its two forms) was again grouped with catatonia and *dementia paranoides*, but the group heading now read Idiot-Producing Processes, instead of Degenerating Psychological Processes. And, whereas in the fourth edition the tripartite group had stood as an equal with twelve other diagnostic categories, it was now demoted to a subordinate position within the category, Metabolic Diseases. Also included in that category were myxedema and cretinism (both caused by low levels of thyroid hormone), and *dementia paralytica* (caused by a bacterium). By moving *dementia praecox*, catatonia and *dementia paranoides* into Metabolic Diseases, Kraepelin confirmed his belief that all three diseases were caused by toxins.

–//–

In the last year of the nineteenth century, Kraepelin published the sixth edition of his textbook. At nearly one thousand pages in length (original edition), it was much longer than any of its predecessors. He was to publish two more editions in his lifetime, adding another 4418 pages for an aggregate total of 8422 pages, but the sixth was the most important of all. Its confident tone, engaging observational data and many innovations struck a chord that still resonates today. It was the crowning – albeit controversial – achievement of nineteenth century psychiatry and a cornerstone of modern psychiatry.

The work was published in two volumes. Volume 1 is titled General Psychiatry; it concerns subjects applicable to all mental illnesses. Volume 2, Clinical Psychiatry, is devoted to classification. Near the beginning of the second volume, Kraepelin placed a list of forty-four contemporary textbooks written by other authors, of which fourteen are identified by title. None of these works, however, is discussed in the text. There a few references to journal articles but, on the whole, this is not an academic work. Rather, as stated in the subtitle, it is a practical guide "for students and physicians".

The textbook contains comprehensive accounts of all known mental disorders. Each one is described according to its psychological, behavioral and physical symptoms. More interesting for the non-specialist are Kraepelin's comments in the two Introductions (one for each volume). In Volume 1, he spells out his purposes and methods. For readers who might be in doubt about what psychiatry is, he states unequivocally, in the very first sentence, that "psychiatry is the science of mental illnesses and their treatment." The key word in that sentence is *science*. Having thus made clear his central stance, he goes on to reiterate many points for which he had already become known. For example, he acknowledges the potential of pathological anatomy, but says that it has "so far furnished rather little information." As for what psychology might contribute, his assertion echoes Wilhelm Wundt,

> It is not impossible, with the help of that young science, to create a physiology of the mind capable also of furnishing a useful basis for psychiatry. On the one hand, it can be used for breaking down complex phenomena into their simple constituents ... and we shall also be able, in suitable cases, to directly use the psychologic experiment as a means for a detailed investigation of pathologic conditions ... On the other hand, scientific psychology is likely to provide useful additions to our view on the

> causes of insanity. Here we again have to refer to toxins acting
> upon the course of our mental processes ...[123]

Having opened the Introduction by stating that psychiatry is the science of mental illness, he returns to that key opinion at the very end.

> Psychiatry is a young, still developing science, that must, against sharp opposition, gradually achieve the position it deserves according to its scientific and practical importance. There is no doubt that it will achieve this position – for it has at its disposal the same weapons which have served the other branches of medicine so well: clinical observation, the microscope and experimentation.[124]

Those words ring as true today as they did when written in 1899.

Volume 2 begins with a critique of current practices in respect to classification, emphasizing once again his devotion to the "essential" features of mental disorders.

> By far the most frequently adopted approach to the classification of mental disorders has been to classify them according to their *clinical symptoms*, because it is the manifestations of insanity that most directly strike the eye of the beholder. This procedure ... very soon encounters difficulties, once it becomes a question of distinguishing the essential from the coincidental and nonessential.

Kraepelin then summarizes his own approach, which stresses the connection between diagnosis and prognosis,

> The clinical grouping of psychic disorders will have to be supported *simultaneously* by all three means of classification [pathological anatomy, causation, symptoms], to which must also be added the experiences acquired from the course, the outcome, even the treatment of the disease ... Precisely this procedure is the only one which, at the present stage of development of our science, is also able to some extent to satisfy the *practical* requirements that we have. The first thing the doctor

---

[123]E. Kraepelin (1899, 1990), vol. 1, p. 5.
[124]E. Kraepelin (1899, 1990), vol. 1, p. 8.

has to do at the patient's bedside is form an opinion about the prospective further development of the case of disease. This is always the first question put to him. For the practical activity of the clinician, the value of every diagnosis is thus rated essentially by *the extent to which it opens up reliable prospects for the future* [italics in original].[125]

Dementia praecox is given much greater prominence in this edition than in preceding ones, and it is classified somewhat differently. Whereas *dementia praecox* was grouped with catatonia and *dementia paranoides* in the fourth and fifth editions, it stands alone in the sixth edition as one of thirteen major categories. All the major categories are divided into smaller groupings. *Dementia praecox* has three "forms": hebephrenic, catatonic and paranoid. By way of explanation, Kraepelin wrote, "The first one is identical with the *dementia praecox* which I described earlier, the second with catatonia, and the third embraces *dementia paranoides*."

Another example of a category with multiple types is General Neuroses. Kraepelin includes under this heading three types: epileptic insanity, hysteric insanity and fright neurosis. It is surprising that Kraepelin would use the old term, epileptic insanity, and that he would designate it as a neurosis, given the post-Feuchtersleben definition of neurosis as a purely mental disorder, but he did. Moreover, he lists epileptic dementia and alcoholic epilepsy as subtypes of epileptic insanity.

The clinical description of *dementia praecox* extends to seventy-eight pages. By comparison, Kraepelin needed only ten pages to cover the same subject in the fourth edition, and thirty-nine pages in the fifth edition. His coverage of the disorder is replete with page after page of wild behaviors and bizarre delusions. The inclusion of so much symptom description is surprising, given that the Introduction eschews diagnosis by symptoms. Perhaps he, like previous authors, knew the titillating effect of such material. On the other hand, there are plenty of statistics. Between ten and eleven percent of cases of *dementia praecox* are preceded by a "severe acute illness". Seventeen percent of the individuals in the Heidelberg clinic were "outstandingly talented," and eighteen percent of the women had "menstrual disorders". Seventy-five percent of cases exhibiting the hebephrenic form "appear to reach the higher grades of dementia," whereas seventeen percent continue with "moderate" dementia. As for the remaining eight

---

[125]E. Kraepelin (1899, 1990), vol. 2, pp. 3-4.

percent, "the signs of the hebephrenic disorder vanished so completely that it might be justifiable to speak of recovery."

When addressing the causes of *dementia praecox*, Kraepelin states that a "hereditary predisposition" was found in "seventy percent of those cases in which utilizable data were available," meaning evidence from family members. The disorder, he writes, is "like a tree whose roots no longer find nurture in the available soil, so the intellectual powers are said to dwindle once the inadequate heritage no longer permits further development." It can be noted that Kraepelin's estimate of seventy percent for hereditary predisposition stands remarkably close to the current estimate of eighty percent, which comes from sophisticated statistical analyses.[126]

$$-//-$$

With the identification and elaboration of *dementia praecox*, Kraepelin built one pillar of his reputation. With the identification of manic-depressive insanity in the sixth edition (later named bipolar disorder), he erected a second pillar. Together, these two disorders re-defined the psychoses. Recall that psychosis refers to illnesses which are caused by brain abnormalities. In 1845, when Feuchtersleben defined the term, the abnormalities that were supposed to characterize the psychoses were, for the most part, imagined. Only progressive paralysis left telltale marks in the brain. In 1893, when Kraepelin named *dementia praecox*, progressive paralysis was still the only psychosis with a known neuropathology, and nothing had changed by the time that Kraepelin introduced manic-depressive insanity. Despite the lack of anatomical evidence, Kraepelin took the bold and largely successful step of splitting the entire gamut of psychosis into two neat categories, *dementia praecox* and manic-depressive insanity.

A common, and not incorrect, view of Kraepelin's classification is that it separates disorders of affect (manic-depressive insanity) from disorders of intelligence (*dementia praecox*). In psychiatric parlance, affect refers to a person's mood or emotion – excitement, depression, anxiety, et cetera – while intelligence refers to rationality.

People generally expect and tolerate *variable* affect, but *disorders* of affect were hardly noticed by early psychiatrists. More feared, and therefore more prominent, was the prospect of irrationality. Virtually all mental

---

[126]Ronald Chase, *Schizophrenia: A Brother Finds Answers in Biological Science.* Baltimore, Johns Hopkins University Press (2013), pp. 19-21.

disturbances were considered disorders of intelligence. Prior to the nineteenth century, even melancholy was thought to be a disorder of intelligence. Opinions began to change in the early 1800s under the influence of faculty psychology and romanticism. Johann Heinroth, the religiously minded psychiatrist from Leipzig, was particularly insightful. He dismissed the idea that depression is caused by a faulty intellect, emphasizing instead the role of "disposition" and a "depressing passion".

> It is obviously nonsensical to keep brooding on the imaginary misfortunes of others; but the question is if the true origin of fixed ideas is indeed the intellect, as many are wont to believe. We say: no! In our view this is the false idea of which humanity has held for several hundreds of years ... that the origin of the false notions of patients suffering from melancholia ... is being erroneously attributed to the intellect ... It is the disposition which is seized by some depressing passion.[127]

Meanwhile, mainstream physicians in France were also reevaluating the role of affect in psychiatry. Phillipe Pinel distinguished two types of mania, those involving intelligence (*manie avec délire*) and those that involving mood (*manie sans délire*). Jean-Etienne Esquirol came up with lypemania, a disorder characterized by sadness. With time, mania and depression came to take on their modern meanings, and by mid-century some psychiatrists were noting that mania and depression could appear as an alternating pair in the same patient. It became apparent that mania and depression, while seemingly very different, must have a common origin. Even the names of newly recognized disorders reflected the intimate association between elevated moods and depressed moods, for example, *dysthymia mutablilis*, *la folie circulaire* and *la folie à double forme*.

Two Parisians alienists, Jean-Pierre Falret and Jules Baillarger, had been independently caring for patients with alternating moods. Each of them noted that none of these patients ever became demented. This was an important observation because everyone knew that disorders of intelligence could – and often did – lead to dementia. So, if disorders of mood did *not* lead to dementia, they must be very different from intellectual disorders. Around the same time, Ewald Hecker and Karl Kahlbaum also became interested in mood disorders, due to their pronounced temporal features. Hecker coined the term cyclothymia for a type of recurrent, affective insanity. A few years later, Kahlbaum published his own account

---

[127] J. C. Heinroth (1818, 1975), pp. 190-191.

of the same disorder. In contrast to Hecker, who saw cyclothymia as a true psychosis, Kahlbaum considered it as a relatively mild disorder with a favorable course. Taken together, all these early accounts of mood disorders provided Kraepelin with plenty of precedent for his manic-depressive insanity, just as there had been precedents for *dementia praecox*.

With manic-depressive insanity, Kraepelin achieved what he had promised in his inaugural lecture at Dorpat: the identification of a disorder based on "the *clinical* study of mental disorders, or the empirical determination of individual forms of madness according to their cause, course, and conclusion." In other words, he combined an analysis of symptoms with an analysis of temporal course, and he did so with manic-depressive insanity even more powerfully than he had with *dementia praecox*. Kraepelin's succinct definition of his new illness acknowledges both elements,

> Manic-depressive insanity ... comprises the entire domain of so-called *periodic and circular insanity* on the one hand, and *simple mania* which is usually still distinguished from it, on the other. Over the years, I have convinced myself more and more that all of the described pictures are simply manifestations of a single pathological process ... Manic-depressive insanity takes place in single attacks which present either the signs of a so-called *manic excitation*, flight of ideas, elated mood and urge to be active, or those of a peculiar *psychic depression with psychomotor inhibition*, or finally, a *mixture of the two states.* [italics in original].[128]

By way of further elaboration, he describes how the intensity of the symptoms fluctuates over time, and how each episode is typically interrupted by a "more or less complete return to presence of mind." Since manic-depressive insanity is a form of psychosis, patients in all three states (manic, depressive and mixed) experience delusions. During the manic state, for example,

> The mood is predominately elated and cheerful, and affected by the feeling of increased fitness. The patient feels the need to come out of his shell, to have livelier relations with those around him, to play a role ... The patient establishes many contacts, suddenly pays all this business debts without constraint, makes

---

[128]E. Kraepelin (1899, 1990), vol. 2, p. 272.

magnificent presents, builds all kinds of castles in the air and throws himself with rash enthusiasm into daring ventures that overreach his strength by far. He has 167,000 picture postcards of his village printed, tries to adopt a little black boy from the Cameroon.

Contrastingly, in the depressive state,

The mood is gloomy. Nothing can arouse his interest for long; nothing gives him pleasure; he has become indifferent towards his relatives and to what used to be dearest to him. Everywhere he sees only the drawbacks and difficulties; the people around him are not as good and unselfish as he thought they were; one deception and disillusion follows another." [129]

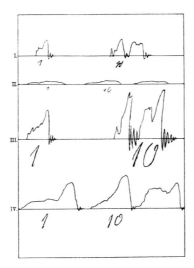

Figure 27: Handwriting in a healthy person (panel I) and in patients with manic-depressive insanity (panels II-IV). [Kraepelin, 1899]

According to Kraepelin, "By far the most striking disturbances [in manic-depressive insanity] lie in the psychomotor domain." He was referring to abnormalities in his patients' physical movements. To illustrate the point,

---

[129] E. Kraepelin (1899, 1990), vol. 2. Manic and depressive states described respectively on pp. 285 and 293.

he reproduced experimental data from his Heidelberg laboratory (Figure 27).

Patients were asked to write the numbers 1 and 10. They used a special stylus that recorded the quickness of their finger movements and the amount of pressure that was applied to the paper. Panel number I (at the top) is a control, taken from a "healthy female guard". The speed and pressure tracing is above the line, the actual writing below. Panel II is from a manic-depressive patient in a depressive state. The numbers are smaller than in panel I, the speed of writing is "greatly retarded", and the pressure is "not even 50 grams." Panel III is from a manic-depressive patient in a manic state. "It may be considered as the expression of the intensified psychomotor excitability." Finally, panel IV is from a woman who "was in a condition where the urge to be active had vanished completely for a few days in the course of severe mania." Panel IV, therefore, represents the mixed state.

Kraepelin presents *dementia praecox* and manic-depressive insanity in separate chapters. Although he gives us lengthy descriptions of the symptoms associated with each illness, there is little in the way of direct comparison. To fill the gap, I made my own comparison using statistics that Kraepelin left scattered throughout the text (Figure 28). These percentages indicate a surprising similarity in quantifiable aspects of the illnesses.

	Dementia praecox	Manic-depressive Insanity
Prevalence in the clinic	14 - 15%	10 - 15%
Females	36% in hebephrenic form 58% in catatonic form 59% in paranoid form	66%
Age of onset under 25 years	60%	66%
Hereditary cause	80%	70%

Figure 28: Statistical comparison of *dementia praecox* and manic-depressive insanity. Author's tabulation, based on percentages reported in Kraepelin's textbook (1899].

Moreover, Kraepelin provides little practical guidance for distinguishing *dementia praecox* from manic-depressive insanity during diagnosis.

> The depressive states [of manic-depressive insanity] have to be distinguished, above all, from the introductory depression of

> *dementia praecox* ... the emphasis here lies on the distinction
> between negativism and psychomotor inhibition, which can be
> very difficult in the given case. Also to be taken into consid-
> eration are the presence of mind and the absence of thought
> disturbance, and also particularly the emotional dullness in *de-
> mentia praecox*, as opposed to the hebetude [lethargy], absence
> of mind and sad or anxious depression in the case of [manic-
> depressive insanity]. Rapid occurrence of very nonsensical delu-
> sional ideas and numerous illusions without marked clouding of
> the consciousness and depression speaks very much for *dementia
> praecox.*[130]

Psychiatrists would have had to cull the essence of each disorder from
the totality of material provided in Kraepelin's textbook. Once distilled,
it came down to two distinguishing features. First, *dementia praecox* is
fundamentally a disturbance of rational thought, whereas manic-depression
is a disturbance of mood. And second, *dementia praecox* progresses to
dementia, but manic-depressive insanity does not.

–//–

As the diseases named by his predecessors faded from memory, it was Kraepelin's terminology and Kraepelin's classification that stood tall. Gone
were the empty speculations of the past, Heinroth's romantic psychiatry
and Gudden's indifference to diagnosis. Kraepelin ruled with the authority of science and the persuasion of fact-filled writing. Here at last was a
natural order suited to a modern psychiatry. So the story goes, but there
are more nuanced versions, as we will see.

No one denies that the sixth edition of Kraepelin's textbook is a master-
piece. It is actually unique in many respects, for it contains not only the
robust case descriptions for which Kraepelin is renown, but also many sup-
plementary materials of a more scientific nature. He includes photographs
to illustrate the body types and facial features supposedly typical of particular illnesses. There are group portraits of individuals diagnosed with
the same illness, such as the photograph of catatonic patients reproduced
on page 170 of this book. Mood states in manic-depression are illustrated
with multiple photographs of the same patient. Two photographic plates
show histological changes in the cerebral cortex, one of which is credited to
Nissl.

---

[130]E. Kraepelin (1899, 1990), vol. 2, p. 318-319.

Kraepelin also took full advantage of mechanical recording devices to illustrate abnormal motor behaviors. Figure 27, showing the numbers 1 and 10 written by a manic-depressive patient, is one example. He has thirteen additional "specimens" of his patients' handwriting, each containing several lines of script. And impressively, he presents quantitative data in graphs. There are graphs showing the ages of illness onset, body weights over time, and the ups and downs of symptoms such as melancholy, stupor and agitation. All of these illustrations – photographs, physiological traces, graphs – are examples of scientific methodology. Kraepelin did not forsake clinical symptoms, he sought to objectify them with measurements and statistics. In this respect, with varying degrees of success, he replaced personal observation with "hard facts". And, in so far as objective data are superior to subjective opinions for purposes of defining and diagnosing diseases, these innovations were a step forward.

It is generally assumed that Kraepelin took his quantitative data from the *Zählkarten*, the cards on which he and his assistants recorded details of the patients' medical histories. Although he may well have extracted information from the cards pertaining to ages, family profiles and disease outcomes, the more interesting question is the extent to which he used the cards for constructing his classification. According to one of Kraepelin's students, he "again and again worked through thousands and thousands of his patients' files in order to group and re-group them."[131]

One can imagine Kraepelin sitting at his desk in the bungalow behind his house. Stacks of *Zählkarten* lie neatly arranged on the desktop, some tall, some short. There is a stack for progressive paralysis, one for *dementia praecox*, others for idiocy, hysteria, alcoholism and so on. Many more cards lay strewn about, these not yet assigned to any stack. Kraepelin picks up one of the loose cards and reads from it. The patient is a male. He was admitted to the clinic at age twenty-three and is described as "unkempt". His mother suffers from depression, his father is an alcoholic. The patient's speech is disorganized, his behavior "agitated". An assistant physician has noted the patient's stiff, somewhat lopsided movements. In which stack should Kraepelin place the card ? He holds it before him, hovering between *dementia praecox* and manic-depressive insanity. Then he notices that this patient is no longer in the clinic. Two years previously, his condition had been characterized as "demented" and he was sent to the asylum

---

[131] Quoted in Matthias M. Weber and Eric J. Engstrom, "Kraepelin's 'diagnostic cards': the confluence of clinical research and preconceived categories," *History of Psychiatry* 8:375-385 (1997), p. 383.

at Heppenheim. There is no longer any question. Kraepelin puts the card on the *dementia praecox* stack and turns to another unsorted card.

According to one historian,

> [The] crucial distinction from Kahlbaum and Hecker – and Kraepelin's major contribution – was that he had detailed, quantifiable data collected longitudinally over a period of years. No one had ever approached the identification ... of the insanities using a structured scientific method ... [It was] systematic science.[132]

Other authors have disputed these claims, at least in respect to Kraepelin's reliance on the *Zählkarten*. Two historians of German psychiatry, Matthias Weber and Eric Engstrom, examined a collection of 705 *Zählkarten* kept in the archives of the Max-Planck-Institute of Psychiatry in Munich.[133] Although Kraepelin ended his career in Munich, most of the cards in the institute's collection date from his earlier years in Heidelberg. According to Weber and Engstrom, notations on the cards are written using "commonplace expressions of everyday speech," rather than precise clinical terminology. There is "a lack of systematic rigor, and [the use of] incomplete diagnostic terms." Furthermore, it is apparent that individual patients were followed, on average, for only around three months, far less than would be required for a meaningful assessment of disease outcomes. And most damaging for the claim that the cards were used for sorting illnesses by outcomes, "more than 54% of the cards do not give any information about the course of the disease."

In discussing the implications of their investigation, Weber and Engstrom quote from one of Kraepelin's last published articles (1919). There, he admits that the cards were a "means of last resort" and that the patients' case reports had to be condensed so as to represent the "important" facts. Weber and Engstrom contend that any such condensation would have been influenced by preconceived notions of what the facts of a case *should* be. If, for example, Kraepelin suspected that an individual might be suffering from manic-depressive insanity, his assessment of that patient would be biased toward memories of his or her emotional states. Weber and Engstrom conclude that Kraepelin's understanding of disease entities may well have been acquired "outside, before, or perhaps despite his clinical observations."

---

[132]Richard Noll, *American Madness: The Rise and Fall of Dementia Praecox*. Cambridge, MA, Harvard University Press (2011), p. 63.

[133]M. M. Weber and E. J. Erickson (1997).

Thus, "Kraepelin's concept of diagnosis and prognosis was to a considerable degree a theoretical ideal which cannot be easily verified on the basis of his clinical case records."

Taking all of this into account, it would seem that Kraepelin did try to use quantitative methods, but he fell short of modern standards in respect to design and implementation. The questionable value of the *Zählkarten* reminds one of the dubious quantitation in his pharmacological and psychological experiments. In balance, perhaps it would be fair to say that Kraepelin's classification was as much the product of his insights as it was his objective methods of data collection.

–//–

History has shown that the sixth edition was a huge success. Kraepelin probably anticipated the result, because he got it into the hands of booksellers just in time for the new state examinations in psychiatry. Two years later, flush with the money earned from its sales, he bought a parcel of land at Suna near Pallanza, Italy, upon which he built a beautiful vacation villa.

Immediately after completing the manuscript, in the Spring of 1899, Kraepelin and his brother traveled to Egypt. It was a vacation well deserved by Emil and long awaited by both men. They began their trip in Cairo where "almost all the guests in [the] hotel were Germans ... We were particularly impressed by the mule drivers." A few days later, they took a saloon-train to Luxor, where they viewed royal graves, ruins and ancient monuments. After a steamboat ride to Aswan, they returned to Cairo. They made excursions in and around the city, visited museums, carpet bazaars and other local attractions. Emil then visited a mental asylum, because he "was particularly interested in seeing some of the mental disorders caused by hashish." After the visit, "with Professor Dinkler's assistance, [he] succeeded in acquiring a large lump of hashish to take home." He was disappointed, one supposes, when he experienced "no distinct effects" from smoking the drug.[134]

Kraepelin was back in Germany by autumn, and probably in Heidelberg at the end of the year, which was the final year of the nineteenth century. New Year's Eve, known as Silvester in Germany, was always celebrated, but this year's New Year's Eve was special. One imagines Kraepelin in his home on *Scheffelstraße*, logs burning slowly in the fireplaces. The girls –

---

[134]Quotes from Kraepelin (1987), pp. 91-94.

Antonie, Eva, Ina and Hanna – would have been allowed to stay up late so as to witness the magical moment. One can picture Emil and Ina welcoming their guests, he dressed in a dark suit buttoned high on a starched white shirt with bow tie, Ina in a white silk gown flaring like a trumpet at the ankle and tight (with corset) at the waist. The expectant crowd was no doubt offered plenty of French Champagne and *Glühwein*, but Emil would have had none of that. He was drinking *Apfelsaft*.

With the sound of bells ringing throughout the city, fireworks exploded above the brown rooftops along the Neckar river. The American author, Mark Twain, would have recognized the scene. Visiting in Heidelberg on an earlier occasion, he described "meteor showers of rockets, Roman candles, bombs, serpents, and Catharine wheels ... discharging in wasteful profusion into the sky."[135]

Two days after that special night, an article in the *Heidelberger Tageblatt* described the celebration.

> Although the Silvester night was pretty noisy, the noise was not a considerable degree greater than in previous years. According to the police report, the protection team had many occasions to intervene, with no shortage of accidents caused by careless handling of fireworks and missiles. A room fire was still burning in the morning. A doctor had to treat as many as five persons injured on Silvester night.

The Kraepelin home provided the perfect view. Looking out from the south-facing windows, Emil would have seen the city illuminated, and above it the castle ruins brooding darkly. Not immune to the significance of the occasion, he must have felt deeply satisfied. It had been a good year for him, and a good century for psychiatry.

---

[135]Mark Twain, *A Tramp Abroad*. Charleston, Bibliolife (1880, 2007), appendix B.

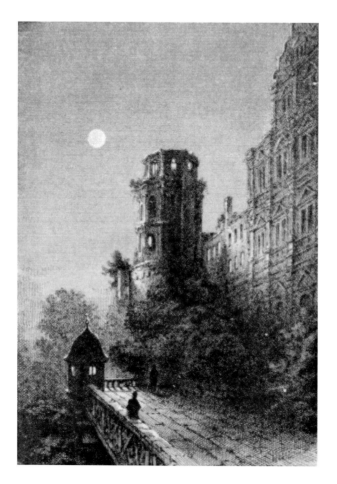

Figure 29: The Schloss at Heidelberg. [Mark Twain, 1880]

16 Nineteenth Century Psychiatry Today and in the Future

History is continuous, so changing the calendar from the nineteenth century to the twentieth century did not affect the development of psychiatry. It did, however, end the narrative of this book. In the final chapter, I will review and reflect upon nineteenth century psychiatry from the vantage point of the early twenty-first century.

Johann Christian Reil coined the word psychiatry in 1808. At the time, patients with obvious mental symptoms were housed together with physically ill patients in poorly funded asylums that offered little in the way of basic comforts, let alone treatment. The attending physicians thought the patients mad, but knew not the types, the causes, nor even the words with which to describe the maladies.

One hundred years later – by the early twentieth century – psychiatry was a full-fledged medical specialty. Its practitioners understood that the mind, the brain and behavior are all intimately linked. Patients were generally well cared for, even if there were few effective treatments. And, the intellectual basis of psychiatric practice, which had been shaky just fifty years earlier, was now secure. Thanks to the ideas of Wilhelm Griesinger, Karl Kahlbaum and Emil Kraepelin, the major mental illnesses were identified and classified, and a course was charted toward understanding their neurobiological bases.

We are now more than two hundred years removed from Reil's neologism, and more than one hundred years past Kraepelin's sixth edition textbook. We need to ask, How many of the specific ideas from the nineteenth century remain valid today? Which ones have been modified? Which ones discarded? I will answer these questions by examining four assertions, which together summarize what are considered to be the major achievements of nineteenth century psychiatry. I will look separately at each assertion, noting events from the twentieth and twenty-first centuries that bear on the its current relevance. Along the way, I will express some personal opinions about the issues raised, and even be so bold as to predict the future of scientific psychiatry.

Assertion No. 1: Mental illness is an illness

The English term *mental illness* is relatively new, dating from 1847, when the novelist Emily Brontë used it in chapter fourteen of her novel, *Wuthering Heights.* She wrote, "I thought, too, it might create a favorable crisis in Catherine's mental illness ..." In the same year, Emily's Brontë's older sister, Charlotte, wrote in her novel, *Jane Eyre*, of a fictional character who had *mental defects.* What exactly did the authors mean by these terms?

Most likely, the Brontë sisters were writing with metaphorical intent. They would not have referenced a mental illness in the sense that we use that term today, because the medical model for psychiatry had not yet been established. It would be another two or three decades before that concept took hold. Wilhelm Griesinger introduced the medical model at the Charité hospital in Berlin, Kraepelin adopted it in Heidelberg, and Kraepelin further refined it after moving to Munich in 1903.

The University Psychiatric Clinic in Munich occupied a magnificent new building. It had one hundred beds divided among nine wards, a large out-patient department, a microscopy laboratory and a library. The clinic operated as a modern hospital, meaning that research went hand-in-hand with patient care. Alois Alzheimer moved to Munich along with Kraepelin, and Franz Nissl joined them later. In addition to neuroanatomy, physician-scientists in Munich pursued research in experimental psychology, physiology, blood chemistry and heredity.

Before his death, in 1926, Kraepelin cemented his legacy as a champion of biological psychiatry by creating the German Institute for Psychiatric Research, which later became the Max Planck Institute of Psychiatry. World-class clinical care and basic research continues to this day in the buildings first occupied by Kraepelin and colleagues. Only the street address has changed. Whereas the clinic was built on *Nussbaumstraße*, it now sits on *Kraepelinstraße*.

While Kraepelin was pursuing his vision of a scientific psychiatry in Munich, Sigmund Freud was developing a very different approach in Vienna. Some people have taken the disagreement to mean that Freud did not believe in the medical model, but this is untrue. It was just that his medical model differed from Kraepelin's. Whereas Kraepelin built his on biological principles, Freud relied on psychology. Nevertheless, and despite the fact that most psychiatrists lined up with one or the other leader throughout the twentieth century, the men themselves had much in common and their ideas were in many ways complementary. Freud, like Kraepelin, was a fully qualified medical doctor. While it is true that Freud treated patients in his home and had no affiliation with any clinic or hospital, he insisted that his disciples receive conventional medical training.

Kraepelin and Freud were both born in the year 1856, and both were German speaking, but they traveled parallel paths, with only a single significant crossing. Although each man was aware of the other's work, there is no evidence of any correspondence. Kraepelin did not see Freud when he visited Vienna, and Freud may never have visited Germany.[136] Their personal relationship may have been tenuous, but it was neither bitter nor competitive.

Early in his career, Freud spent a few months with Theodor Meynert, a highly respected neuroanatomist. Then he then went to Paris where he worked with Jean-Martin Charcot, a neurologist who was experimenting with hypnosis as a treatment for hysteria. Charcot considered hysteria to be a disorder of the nervous system, but Freud thought otherwise, and thus began Freud's pivot into psychiatry.

Freud's psychiatric career played out mostly after 1900. Here, I will briefly summarize its substance, insofar as it relates to Kraepelin and nineteenth century psychiatry. Soon after leaving Paris, and with the conversations with Charcot fresh in mind, Freud co-authored *Studies on Hysteria*, published in 1895. In this book, Freud introduced several seminal ideas that later formed the basis of psychoanalysis, his psychological approach to the treatment of mental illness. He wrote, among other things, that hysteria is not a brain abnormality, but a disorder caused by a psychological defense mechanism. He discarded Charcot's hypnosis in favor of a new therapeutic technique, which he called "free association". Freud's patients were encouraged to open their minds and speak "freely" about what they were thinking.

Kraepelin learned of Freud's interpretation of hysteria while preparing the sixth edition of his textbook. In a section dealing with hysteria, Kraepelin commented sardonically on Freud's views,

> According to their assertions [Freud and Joseph Breuer] hysteria is caused by specific passive sexual experiences in earliest childhood, which then continue to haunt the individual during his whole life ... But if our much troubled mind really loses its equilibrium forever due to long forgotten unpleasant sexual

---

[136]Nowhere in the biographies of Sigmund Freud have I found evidence of any travel to Germany. There are, however, many biographies that I have not read.

experiences, it would seem that we have reached the beginning
of the end of mankind; nature would have played a cruel hoax
on us![137]

Also in 1895, Freud wrote an essay titled *Project for a Scientific Psychology*. It is a short, theoretical work that addresses brain mechanisms possibly responsible for certain psychological phenomena. Thus, it is more aligned with Kraepelin's interests than his book on hysteria. Although the work was left unfinished, and not published until long after his death, it was eventually praised for its farsightedness. Freud was obviously well acquainted with the work of Ramón y Cajal, and in the essay he clearly endorses what he calls "the theory of neurons". Speculating on the means of communication between neurons, he proposes the existence of "contact barriers", which could be adjusted to allow for variable degrees of communication. Such an arrangement, he wrote, could provide a physical substrate for memories. Remarkably, research completed many decades later demonstrated the reality of neuronal synapses, and later still, research demonstrated that human memories reside in structurally modified synapses. Thus, both of Freud's conjectures have been proven essentially correct.

Laying aside the incomplete *Project*, Freud turned his attention to psychoanalysis. In 1900, one year after Kraepelin's sixth edition textbook, Freud published *The Interpretation of Dreams*, which was the first of his fully psychoanalytic writings. The contrast between Kraepelin's textbook and Freud's *Dreams* is striking. Clearly, Kraepelin and Freud were at odds about the nature of mental illness and the relevance of psychology to psychiatry. Kraepelin thought of psychology in terms of Wundt's mental processes. For him, the deep structures of the mind were fundamentally the same in everyone – healthy subjects as well as mentally ill persons. Freud's understanding of psychology, by contrast, was focused on the unique inner conflicts of disturbed individuals. In a similar vein, Kraepelin assumed that mental illnesses develop either from hereditary defects or when toxins affect the brain, whereas Freud looked upon them as arising from the patient's subjective experiences. It has been said that Kraepelin sought to discover diseases, whereas Freud sought to understand personalities.

The only squabble directly involving Freud and Kraepelin came about after a German judge named Daniel Schreber published a memoir about his own psychotic illness. (Schreber, who was briefly treated by Kraepelin's irritable boss, Paul Flechsig, described Flechsig as the "murderer

---

[137]E. Kraepelin (1899, 1990), pp. 381-382.

of my soul.") Freud identified Schreber's disorder as *dementia paranoides*, in accordance with Kraepelin's classification, but he interpreted the case differently than Kraepelin. Freud wrote that Schreber's illness originated in his boyhood homosexual desires. To defend himself against the unwanted thoughts, Schreber had unconsciously "repressed" them. Accordingly, Freud saw Schreber's illness as a conflict between his sex drive and his ego. Kraepelin bought none of that. For him, Schreber's paranoia was caused by a biological process that was likely rooted in a hereditary disposition.

Freud developed his ideas in Vienna, and came to America only once, in 1909, to deliver a series of five lectures at Clark University in Worchester, Massachusetts. Adolf Meyer, the outspoken critic of Nissl's fibril theory, also spoke at the Clark conference. Although Meyer had spent time with Kraepelin in Europe, and had endorsed his ideas, he now abandoned Kraepelin in favor of Freud. His enthusiastic support of Freud's ideas secured a huge following for Freud in America. American psychiatrists welcomed psychoanalysis as a panacea for anxieties, "sexual deviations", "nervous breakdowns" and other neuroses (disorders without obvious neurological defects).

The popularity of psychoanalysis, both in American psychiatry and in the public imagination, peaked in the 1950s and 1960s. It was seriously demoted in the third edition of the Diagnostic and Statistical Manual of Mental Disorders (1980), and continued to decline thereafter. Today, it is found almost entirely in the offices of certain psychotherapists who borrow from Freud's ideas and techniques in the treatment of personality disorders. Writing about psychoanalysis in his full-length history of psychiatry, Edward Shorter refers to it as the "dinosaur ideology of the nineteenth century."

> [I]t was only for a few moments that the patient recumbent upon the couch, the analyst seated silently behind him, occupied the center stage of psychiatry. By the 1970s, the progress of science within psychiatry would dim the lights on this scenario, marginalizing psychoanalysis within the discipline of psychiatry as a whole. In retrospect, Freud's psychoanalysis appears as a pause in the evolution of biological approaches to brain and mind rather than as the culminating event in the history of psychiatry.[138]

---

[138] E, Shorter (1997), quotes on pp. 145 and 170.

Notwithstanding their disagreements, Kraepelin and Freud were united in regarding madness as a form of illness. That uniformity of opinion, combined with the high esteem enjoyed by both men within their respective professional circles, helped to secure a place for psychiatry within medicine. Public opinion accepted the concept of mental illness more slowly, but with time it too fell in line. The consensus threatened to fall apart only in the 1970s when some people started to believe that mental illness is nothing but a myth.

$$-//-$$

Doubts about whether mental conditions are really medical illnesses arose from several sources. One was a study in which eight healthy people were admitted to a hospital after faking a mental condition. Even though they attempted to behave normally once they had been admitted, all were detained for long periods, in one case fifty-two days. People saw the study as evidence that even trained psychiatrists cannot distinguish mental illness from normal oddness. Other studies, of family dynamics, pointed out that even otherwise normal people exhibit extreme behaviors when stressed. And, critics pointed out that judgments of what constitutes insanity have varied greatly throughout recorded history. Even now, diverse opinions persist within and between cultures. If there are no objective criteria, argued the critics, perhaps there is nothing there. All of these arguments, and more, were encapsulated in a highly influential book written by the American psychiatrist Thomas Szasz. Published in 1961 with the unabashed title, *The Myth of Mental Illness*, it carried the message that patients who are identified with mental problems are nothing more than social misfits, the unfortunate victims of scapegoating and maltreatment.

The authors of these critiques were not uninformed cranks, but well-intended psychiatrists and academics who challenged the very meaning of the word "illness" and its equivalent, "disease".[139] They made two kinds of claims. Some authors said that only physical conditions can be illnesses.

---

[139] "*Illness* is generally used as a synonym for *disease*. However, this term is occasionally used to refer specifically to the patient's personal experience of his or her disease. In this model, it is possible for a person to have a disease without being ill (to have an objectively definable, but asymptomatic, medical condition, such as a subclinical infection), and to be *ill* without being *diseased* (such as when a person perceives a normal experience as a medical condition, or medicalizes a non-disease situation in his or her life – for example, a person who feels unwell as a result of embarrassment, and who interprets those feelings as sickness rather than normal emotions)." https://www.en.wikipedia.org/wiki/Disease.

Others said that mental conditions may be bad but not sufficiently disabling to be deemed illnesses.

The question of what is, and what is not, an illness, goes back at least to Aristotle. Scholars do not agree upon any particular definition. Illness is commonly understood as a malfunction of a biological organ or process, but most contemporary philosophers think that that definition is too broad. Rachel Cooper, for example, is a specialist in the philosophy of medicine and, in particular, the philosophy of psychiatry. After reviewing several competing accounts of disease, she concludes,

> There is much work to be done with developing an account of disease. However, I suggest that a consensus is emerging with respect to some key issues: first, most of the accounts of disease being developed treat physical and mental disorders together ... Secondly, there is a general consensus that diseases are necessarily harmful.[140]

Cooper adds a further stipulation, namely that a condition must be medically treatable for it to qualify as a disease. Since treatments are now available for most, possibly all, mental conditions, Cooper maintains that mental illnesses pass that final philosophical test. Moreover, few people today give credence to Thomas Szasz's mythical view of mental disorder. Governments, medical institutions, and popular attitudes are – for the most part – comfortable with the idea that mental illness *is* an illness. Whether mental illness is in the mind or in the brain is a separate issue, which I discuss below.

Assertion No. 2: Mental illness is a brain illness

Once again, we can look to the history of words to find clues about how ideas have changed over time. As I have already noted, the word "madness" first appeared in a document dated to 1330 (according to the Oxford English Dictionary). Expressions linking madness to the brain appeared much later. The first documented example is "crack-brained", which was used in 1634. Afterwards, it was not until 1770 that "brainsickly" appeared in print, followed by "mad-brained" in 1822. It would seem, therefore, that

---

[140]Rachel Cooper, *Psychiatry and Philosophy of Science*. Montreal, McGill-Queen's University Press (2007), p. 42.

the notion of mental illnesses as brain illnesses grew slowly through the centuries.

"Patients with so-called mental illnesses are really individuals with illnesses of the nerves and brain," said Wilhelm Griesinger in 1868. Subsequent authors often quoted the statement out of context, turning it into "mental illnesses are brain illnesses," which is shorter, but also stronger. Griesinger – and Kraepelin too – were more cautious. They understood the difference between belief and proof. They knew that brain anatomy was still a young science and that the truly significant findings were yet to come. Be patient, they advised, let the scientists do their work. Meanwhile, disagreements about the fundamental nature of mental illness continued.

The central issue of mind versus brain was kept alive in arguments between the *Psychiker* and the *Somatiker*. It was highlighted in discussions over the definitions of neurosis and psychosis. Then, making matters worse, two new terms were introduced. These were the so-called "organic" illnesses and the so-called "functional" illnesses. Organic was roughly equivalent to psychotic (in the sense of brain-based), and functional was roughly equivalent to neurotic (in the sense of psychological). But, confusion ensued. Lecturing in 1912, one German psychiatrist recalled,

> For a time, 'functional' meant merely that we cannot yet prove anatomical changes with our present day equipment ... Today, however, the adjective is also used in the sense that by such disorders we mean those that will never have a pathological anatomy because they cannot have one.[141]

Even as late as 1978, the well-regarded Swiss psychiatrist, Manfred Bleuler, thought the organic/functional dichotomy useful. He, therefore, referred to senile dementia, progressive paralysis and the psychoses resulting from head trauma as organic illnesses. By contrast, according to Bleuler, schizophrenia and manic-depressive illness were functional disorders, because their biological bases were unknown.

The lack of solid evidence for brain pathologies was a problem for everyone, not to be relieved until the 1970s. Theoreticians were stymied and clinicians frustrated by the absence of biological markers for diagnosis. The anatomists were just plain discouraged. Even Franz Nissl, who had doggedly sought brain correlates for decades, began to despair. When asked

---

[141] German E. Berrios, Rogelio Luque and José M. Villagrán, "Schizophrenia: a conceptual history." *International Journal of Psychology and Psychological Therapy* 3:111-140 (2003), p. 124.

to speak about recent advances in psychiatry at a meeting of the Natural History and Medical Association of Heidelberg, in 1907, he said,

> While we can be proud of our tremendous role in the development of brain anatomy, we cannot ignore the fact that in as much as the studies of brain anatomy have devoured us since the end of the [eighteen] sixties, so clinical psychiatry has been as good as lost ... It was a bad mistake not to realize that the findings of brain anatomy [would bear] no relationship to psychiatric findings, unless the relationships between brain anatomy and brain function were first clarified, and they certainly have not been up to the present.[142]

Nissl went on to say that the focus on anatomy at the expense of clinical psychiatry had given birth to what he called "speculative anatomical teachings", such as in the works of Freud's neuroanatomy mentor, Theodor Meynert. These are disparaging comments, implying that his own research, as well as that of many contemporary anatomists, had been an unproductive sideshow. Not only had it failed to produce anything useful, it had also impeded patient-oriented work.

Ironically, Nissl's comments came in the same year in which the Nobel Prize for Medicine and Physiology was jointly awarded to Santiago Ramón y Cajal and Camillo Golgi for their pioneering work in elucidating the cellular organization of the nervous system. It was – and is – the custom for Nobel laureates to give short speeches describing their work. On this occasion, the two winners famously presented different interpretations of their works. Cajal argued for neuronism (physically separated individual neurons) while Golgi argued for reticularism (all neurons joined in a continuous web). It would be another half-century before unequivocal evidence showed the correctness of Cajal's neuronism (also known as the neuron theory). The resolution of this long-standing controversy fostered an acceleration of neuroscience research.

Much of the anatomical work from the nineteenth century, including some of Nissl's research, remains relevant and valid today. Nissl's aniline dye stains are a mainstay in most neuroanatomy laboratories, and the small granules that he discovered, the "Nissl bodies", are illustrated in nearly every textbook of cell biology. Spinal punctures – so strongly promoted by

---

[142]Franz Nissl, "Über die Entwicklung der Psychiatrie in den letzten 50 Jahren," *Verhandlungen des Naturhistorisch-Medizinischen Vereins*, N.F. 8:510-525 (1908), quote on p. 520.

Nissl – are routinely used in the diagnosis of Alzheimer's disease. Nevertheless, neuroscience in the twenty-first century is very different from what it was in Nissl's time. Neither the methods now available, nor the results obtained using those methods, could have been imagined by Nissl and colleagues. It is now possible, for example, to obtain detailed images of the entire brain in living persons, and even monitor localized brain activity in patients while they engage in assigned tasks. Also, animal models of certain psychiatric illnesses allow researchers to manipulate genes and control neuronal activity, thus enabling strong tests of mechanistic hypotheses.

The powerful methods of modern neuroscience have revealed numerous anatomical, biochemical and physiological features that are, on average, different in the brains of persons with mental illness than in healthy individuals. However, because there is considerable overlap, these findings are not yet useful for diagnosis or treatment.

One particularly well-documented example of an illness-linked biomarker is the size of brain areas. It is now relatively easy to measure brain structures in living patients, thanks to whole brain imaging and computer-assisted analysis. In a study that compared the brains of 2540 healthy persons and 2028 patients with schizophrenia, researchers found that certain areas, including the hippocampus, the amygdala and the thalamus, are considerably smaller in schizophrenia brains than in healthy brains, whereas the opposite is true for other areas, such as the putamen, the pallidum and the lateral ventricle.[143] While a statistical analysis showed that these results are unlikely to have occurred strictly by chance, the extent to which they reflect medication usage or life styles is unsettled.

One of Nissl's cherished goals was to identify function-specific neuron types. He failed because his stains highlighted only a small number of the many physical and chemical properties of nerve cells, and he was unable to relate those particular properties to functions. Today, we have a far greater knowledge of neuron types based on morphological, physiological and chemical criteria. Recent work leans heavily on the biochemical composition of neurons, focusing on neurotransmitters, neurotransmitter receptors and ion channels. Aided by the tools of molecular genetics, investigators use these properties to group neurons into types. Whereas Nissl thought there were five types of neurons, today's scientists tell us that there are more than three hundred types, and some of them are implicated in mental illness.

---

[143]T.G.M. van Erp et al. "Subcortical brain volume abnormalities in 2028 individuals with schizophrenia and 2540 healthy controls via the ENIGMA consortium," *Molecular Psychiatry* 21:547-553 (2016).

For example, the parvalbumin basket cells, found in the cerebral cortex, are implicated in schizophrenia. These neurons ordinarily act by inhibiting the activity of a second type of neuron, the pyramidal cells. In persons with schizophrenia, however, basket cells may be less effective in inhibiting pyramidal cells. Since the pyramidal cells are the only neurons in the cerebral cortex that convey messages over long distances, any errant activity on their part is likely to impact normal functions.[144]

A second of Nissl's fascinations, which he acquired from Bernhard Gudden, was fiber bundles and their pathways. This project, too, found new life in contemporary neuroscience. Altogether, nervous fibers constitute about 60% of the human brain volume. Modern imaging methods allow researchers to view all the major tracts in living persons. Moreover, the physical status of the fibers – healthy or damaged – can be precisely measured using special optical techniques. When researchers compared fibers in psychiatric patients and healthy volunteers, they discovered a significant amount of structural damage in the brains of schizophrenia patients. In a follow-up study, researchers scanned the brains of teenagers living in families with a history of schizophrenia. None of these teenagers was ill at the time of scanning, but some had damaged nerve fibers. It turned out that the teenagers who were free of fiber damage grew into healthy adults, but those who had fiber damage as teenagers developed schizophrenia later.[145] This result implies that fiber damage is a *cause* of schizophrenia rather than a *consequence* or schizophrenia, in other words, it is unlikely due to medication or changes in life styles.

Despite all the wondrous findings of modern neuroscience, some people remain unconvinced that mental illnesses are brain illnesses. The National Alliance on Mental Illness (NAMI) was concerned that the rejection of neurobiological accounts might encourage stigma, so it attempted to persuade holdouts by promoting the motto, "Schizophrenia is a disorder of the brain, caused by problems with brain chemistry and brain structure." The statement, however, did not remain for long on NAMI's website. Perhaps people noticed the apparent contradiction between the namc of the organization and the message contained in the motto. After all, the organization is an alliance on *mental* illness. If the illnesses are *mental*, how can they be

---

[144]David A. Lewis et al. "Cortical parvalbumin interneurons and cognitive dysfunction in schizophrenia," *Trends in Neuroscience* 35:57-67 (2012).

[145]Mark M. Bohlken et al. "Structural brain connectivity as a genetic marker for schizophrenia," *Journal of the American Medical Association Psychiatry* 73:11-19 (2016).

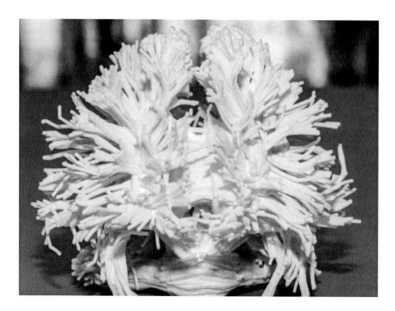

Figure 30: "White matter" in the human brain (posterior view), shown here as a 3-D reconstruction from magnetic resonance diffusion tensor imaging. [Prevue Medical]

caused by *chemistry* and *brain structure*? That question rouses a hornet's nest of philosophical issues.

People who believe in philosophical dualism – whether consciously or unconsciously – have a problem accepting that mental illnesses are brain illnesses. According to the dualistic philosophy, humans possess two types of substances, mind and body. Each is independent of the other, yet each can influence the other. If true, it would follow that the so-called mental illnesses might arise from, and reside in, the mind. Although nearly all academic philosophers disavow dualism as a valid account of mind and consciousness, it remains alive and well in our society.[146]

Public opinion surveys reveal the extent to which people's philosophical beliefs affect their attitudes toward mental illness. For example, in the United States, one survey found that thirty-three percent of the respondents believe that schizophrenia is caused by the patient's "own bad character". In Germany, survey participants were told fictitious stories involving behaviors that mimic those seen in schizophrenia. A striking fifty

---

[146]Ronald Chase, *The Physical Basis of Mental Illness*, New Brunswick, NJ, Transaction (2012).

percent of the respondents cited "lack of will power" as a likely cause of the behaviors. Finally, from a 2008 survey in Canada, forty-six percent of respondents agreed with the statement, "We call some things mental illness because it gives some people an excuse for their poor behavior and personal failing." Ten percent of respondents believed that "most people with mental illnesses could just snap out of it if they really wanted to." This is the stuff of which stigma is made.

Notwithstanding the data noted above, the majority of respondents in recent surveys accept that brain abnormalities underlie mental illness. Many of the same respondents, however, may *also* believe that mental illnesses are in the mind. Dualism allows for such mixed attitudes. The problem is, mixed attitudes contribute to the stigma of mental illness.[147]

Rather than arguing about metaphysics, and possibly promoting stigma in the process, why not avoid the issue entirely? We could take a step in that direction by abandoning the phrase, mental illness, and replacing it with a term like psychiatric illness. Alternatively, we could forego all inclusive terms, replacing them with specialized terms like obsession-compulsion, depression, schizophrenia, et cetera.

Assertion No. 3: *Dementia praecox* (schizophrenia) is a distinct mental illness

Kraepelin did not claim to have discovered *dementia praecox.* He acknowledged the valuable clinical descriptions authored by Karl Kahlbaum, Ewald Hecker and Leon Daraszkiewicz. He knew that similar, if not identical disorders, had already been described and named. It cannot be doubted, however, that Kraepelin put *dementia praecox,* and thus schizophrenia, in the textbooks. There are few other psychiatric disorders from that period that still hold a place in psychiatric classifications. Kraepelin's account of *dementia praecox* drew attention to age of onset as a diagnostic criterion, and it paved the way for the emergence of child psychiatry as a medical specialty. Nevertheless, one needs to ask, how solid is the notion of schizophrenia as an actual disease? As I stated above, a condition of human suffering can qualify as a disease (or illness) even if its symptoms

---

[147]M. C. Angermeyer and S. Dietrich, "Public beliefs about and attitudes towards people with mental illness: a review of population studies," *Acta Psychiatrica Scandinavica* 113:163-179 (2006). For additional survey data and their implications for stigma, see R. Chase (2013), chapter 14.

are predominately mental. The question now is whether schizophrenia is real enough and distinct enough.

Kraepelin spent his entire adult life searching for mental diseases that really exist. According to the Kraepelin scholar, Paul Hoff, who has read most, if not all, of Kraepelin's works, Kraepelin's philosophical outlook was founded on a belief in the "real world". It contains, among other things, mental processes and mental states, and they are the same for everyone whether healthy or sick. Moreover, their existence does not depend on any scientist who might study them. Hoff notes that Kraepelin "often emphasized that the psychiatric researcher has to describe objectively what 'really exists' and what 'nature presents' to him or her." He further states that, "Kraepelin strongly advocated the view that different mental disorders are categorically distinct objects, 'natural kinds' or, as he usually put it, 'natural disease entities'."[148]

Kraepelin's concept of natural disease entities fits with the notion of natural kinds, which has a long history in philosophical literature. While academics debate its exact meaning, most agree that animal species and plant species are natural kinds. Each has its own essence, to use the word favored by Kahlbaum and Kraepelin. Natural kinds of things are "out there" and "real", not simply imagined. Atomic elements are also considered to be natural kinds. Definitions get dicey, however, when it comes to californium and einsteinium, two elements that can be made in the laboratory but are not found in nature. Are they natural kinds? And, what are we to make of animal hybrids, sub-species and "forms"? Although found in nature, these variants beg the question of how distinctive and how stable a thing must be for it to be a natural kind. Charles Darwin taught us to think of biological species as continuously changing. Any given species is capable of changing so much (over a long period of time), that it ceases to be *that* species, but becomes a new one.

Similarly, the history of psychiatry contains the names of numerous mental conditions that were once thought to be "real", but which later turned out to be "unreal". Perhaps the best example is hysteria. The term first appeared in the seventeenth century. In the nineteenth century, it was widely used in clinical descriptions, albeit with variable interpretations. Not until 1980 was it abandoned as a diagnostic term. Its doom was sealed by the absence of any consistent description. At different times, and according to different authorities, hysteria meant a type of epilepsy, a psychosomatic

---

[148]Paul Hoff, "The Kraepelian tradition," *Dialogues in Clinical Neuroscience* 17: 31-41 (2015), quotes on p. 33.

illness, a movement disorder, a personality disorder, and a catchphrase for certain female behaviors unfamiliar to male doctors.

It is not unusual for people to hold inconsistent opinions about what they see and hear. These disagreements may raise concerns, but they do not necessarily imply that the thing in question is other than a natural kind. For thousands of years, people have reported seeing bright objects suddenly appear in the night sky, only to fade away in the following weeks. In China, in the fourth century, one such bright object was described as a "guest star". Observers in sixteenth century Europe thought they were aberrant phenomena associated with the earth's atmosphere. Now we know them as supernovas, and they are a natural kind.

Just as hysteria and supernovas have had different interpretations through time, so too has Kraepelin's concept of d*ementia praecox* been refined, redefined and of course, renamed. Rarely, if ever, has the disorder enjoyed a consensus definition. Does that mean that *dementia praecox*, like hysteria, is not a natural kind of mental illness? Or, does it mean that *dementia praecox*, like supernovas, has finally been correctly defined?

Alfred Hoche, a German psychiatrist known to Kraepelin, did not believe that *dementia praecox* is an illness. He was a unitarian who dismissed the whole idea of conventional psychiatric disorders, claiming that none was truly different from any another. In his opinion, *dementia praecox*, progressive paralysis and senility were all fundamentally the same, all characterized by "progressive disintegration of the mental personality". If they seemed different to some observers, it was only because each one "is accompanied by a colorful palette of symptoms in a great variety of combinations."[149]

Two psychiatrists at the Burgholzli hospital in Zurich decided to take a close look at the symptoms present in their patients diagnosed with *dementia praecox*. They also wanted to find out what became of them over time. Eugen Bleuler and Carl Jung were inquisitive men with a psychoanalytic inclination. They discovered – contrary to Kraepelin's statements and to their own expectations – that not all the *dementia praecox* patients deteriorated steadily or wound up in a deep, irreversible dementia. No patient was ever "cured", but many benefited from a partial recovery or at least a pause in the decline.

Furthermore, after deeply studying the patients' symptoms, Bleuler and Jung came to see them in a different light than had Kraepelin. Here,

---

[149] Alfred Hoche, "The significance of symptom complexes in psychiatry," transl. R.G. Dening and T.R Dening. *History of Psychiatry* ii:334-343 (1912, 1991), quote on p. 340.

Bleuler's ideas proved especially influential, not least because he renamed the illness. In his book, *Dementia praecox or the Group of Schizophrenias* (1911), Bleuler wrote, "I call *dementia praecox* schizophrenia because ... the splitting of the different psychic functions is one of its most important features." Although the book's title implies an equivalence between *dementia praecox* and schizophrenia (the one *or* the other), the preceding statement makes it clear that Bleuler's schizophrenia is different from Kraepelin's *dementia praecox*. Bleuler envisaged fractures separating intelligence, affect and volition, in other words splits between the faculties of mind discussed by Emanuel Kant and the romantic psychiatrists. His diagnosis of schizophrenia is said to have featured four A's: autism, ambivalence, lowered affect and randomized associations. While he acknowledged a role for brain pathology, he emphasized the patients' subjective experiences, at times interpreting psychological symptoms in psychoanalytic terms. In short, while Kraepelin thought of *dementia praecox* as thoroughly biological, Bleuler saw schizophrenia as basically psychological.

Further changes ensued after *dementia praecox* came to America. Richard Noll tells the fascinating story in his book, *American Madness*. Adolf Meyer brought *dementia praecox* to America in 1896, after returning from a six week visit to Kraepelin's clinic in Heidelberg. Meyer, who was born in Switzerland and studied medicine there, moved to the United States while still a young man. Most of his work was done at Johns Hopkins University in Baltimore. While professionally ambitious – and highly successful – he was inconsistent in his thinking. He initially embraced *dementia praecox* as a fine example of biological psychiatry. Later, he adopted a psychological approach and moved away from *dementia praecox*. He infused his writing with Freudian references and encouraged psychotherapy, even for psychotic disorders (in the sense of severe). As his attacks on *dementia praecox* continued, he stopped using that term entirely, switched to schizophrenia, and later spoke only of "schizophrenic reactions".

From 1950 to 1980, approximately, American psychiatrists followed a loose set of criteria in diagnosing schizophrenia. In Noll's words, "Schizophrenia was simply a synonym for severe functional impairment ... a label for grossly impaired persons who could not meet the 'ordinary demands of life'."[150] Meanwhile, according to the International Classification of Diseases (ICD-8), published by the World Health Organization,

---

[150]Richard Noll, *American Madness: The Rise and Fall of Dementia Praecox*. Cambridge, MA, Harvard University Press (2011), p. 274.

schizophrenia was – and still is –defined by bizarre delusions, delusions of control, abnormal affect, hallucinations and disorganized thinking.

The discrepancy between American and international criteria led to striking differences in the rates of diagnosis. During the 1930s, around twenty-five percent of all psychiatric diagnoses in both New York and London were for schizophrenia. By the 1950s, however, the rate had jumped to between sixty and seventy percent in New York, while remaining steady at twenty-five percent in London.

A study was done to see how psychiatrists in New York and London would evaluate the same patient.[151] For this purpose, interviews with eight selected patients were videotaped and shown to psychiatrists in both countries. All participating psychiatrists were asked to diagnose the same interviewed patients. As it turned out, every patient received more diagnoses of schizophrenia from the New York psychiatrists than from the London psychiatrists. One patient got a diagnosis of schizophrenia from eighty-five percent of the New Yorkers, but only seven percent of the Londoners. The study authors concluded, "The New York and London hospital psychiatrists were found ... to differ profoundly in the criteria they set for making the diagnosis of schizophrenia ..."

Meanwhile, the number and character of schizophrenia subtypes kept changing. Kraepelin originally recognized three subtypes (in the sixth edition of his textbook): catatonic, hebephrenic and paranoid. Eugen Bleuler (1911) accepted Kraepelin's three subtypes, but spoke about a wider "group of schizophrenias" that included, among other inventions, "simple schizophrenia" and "latent schizophrenia". By 1913 (in the eighth edition), Kraepelin's trio of subtypes had risen to eleven subtypes. The current edition of the *Diagnostic and Statistical Manual of Mental Disorders* (DSM-5) contains none of these subtypes but does include several related disorders, namely, schizotypal personality disorder, schizophreniform disorder, schizoaffective disorder and "psychotic disorder not otherwise specified".

In 1939, a psychiatrist named Kurt Schneider published a textbook on psychiatric diagnosis that was translated into English in 1959. Following a second delay of two additional decades, Schneider's work brought about a significant change in the clinical definition of schizophrenia. As the director of Kraepelin's Psychiatric Research Institute, Schneider had access to the

---

[151] United States-United Kingdom Cross-National Project, "The diagnosis and psychopathology of schizophrenia in New York and London," *Schizophrenia Bulletin* 11: 80-102 (1974).

records of the Heidelberg Clinic in the years 1900-1925. Because he wanted to include an unambiguous definition of *dementia praecox* in his textbook, he examined these records, noting in particular the symptoms attributed to each patient diagnosed with the illness. He was assisted in this work by Karl Jaspers, who had personally known many of the patients while working as a psychiatrist in Heidelberg. Jaspers later became a prominent existential philosopher.

Schneider distinguished a group of so-called first-rank symptoms and a group of second-rank symptoms, advising that a patient should be diagnosed with schizophrenia if, and only if, he or she shows *any one* of the first-rank symptoms. There were six first-rank symptoms: auditory hallucinations, delusions of being controlled, delusions of having thoughts withdrawn (from the patient), delusions of having thoughts inserted, thought broadcasting, and delusional perception. Schneider's work struck a chord with a group of American psychiatrists who were looking for well-defined, non-Freudian, definitions for psychotic illnesses. These psychiatrists were labeled "neo-Kraepelians", because they favored a medically-oriented, biological approach consistent with Kraepelin's views. When it came time for a revision of the DSM, in 1980, the neo-Kraepelians insisted that schizophrenia be diagnosed on the basis of Schneider's first-rank symptoms. Consequently, beginning with DSM-III, and continuing as recently as DSM-5 (2013), Schneider's first-rank symptoms have been incorporated into the diagnostic criteria, albeit in different ways in each edition. Schneider's first-rank symptoms also form part of the diagnosis for schizophrenia in the current version of the International Classification of Diseases (ICD-10, 1990).

Clearly, the concept of schizophrenia has had a rough ride through its history. German Berrios, an expert on psychotic disorders and their definitions, examined that history in detail. Working with colleagues, he found many changes in schizophrenia's definition over time, but no consistent direction to the changes.[152] Berrios and co-authors assert that Kraepelin, Bleuler, Meyer and Schneider all described different disorders. The various views eventually "converged" onto the current concept of schizophrenia, which is, therefore, a patchwork incorporating several meanings. The situation described by Berrios and co-authors brings to mind Gertrude Steins' remark about her childhood home in Oakland, California. Upon returning to the city late in life, she discovered that "there is no there, there." Is that

---

[152]G. E. Berrios, R. Luque and J. M. Villagrán (2003).

the case with schizophrenia? Has the concept of schizophrenia become so muddled as to be useless?

The DSM is published by the powerful American Psychiatric Association. In preparation for DSM-5, the Association organized a task force to "field test" the diagnostic criteria that had been proposed for the new manual.[153] The test for schizophrenia involved patients at two large psychiatric clinics – one in Canada, one in the United States. Soon after admission, but prior to any diagnosis, the patients were assessed to determine if they had any symptoms suggestive of schizophrenia. If so, the patient was assigned to two experienced psychiatrists (randomly selected from a large pool). The purpose of the field test was to evaluate the reliability of the diagnostic criteria, that is, to see whether the two doctors would arrive at the same diagnosis for the same patient. Therefore, each patient was interviewed twice, once by each psychiatrist, and neither psychiatrist was made aware of the other's diagnosis. Overall, the study found that when two doctors interviewed the same patient they agreed on the diagnosis about eighty-five percent of the time.

Eighty-five percent is a pretty good result. It shows that, for the most part, the psychiatrists participating in the study understood the diagnostic criteria for schizophrenia *as stated in DSM-5*. The fifteen percent of cases in which the doctors disagreed can be attributed to subjective judgements. But, consistency in diagnosis is not the same as proving that schizophrenia is a disease. It means only that the criteria were clearly stated and clearly present (or not) in the majority of cases. The question remains, is a collection of symptoms that includes hallucinations, disorganized speech, reduced emotions, lack of motivation and social dysfunction sufficient to validate schizophrenia as a real illness?

A more convincing case for the "realness" of schizophrenia would be an objective measurement akin to the blood sugar test for diabetes. Kraepelin thought that he had an objective criterion when he announced that *dementia praecox* invariably went downhill to permanent dementia. People called it "diagnosis by prognosis", but it was a logical nonstarter, and anyway, Bleuler's experience contradicted Kraepelin's. Subsequent observations, including some by Kraepelin himself, confirmed the variable course of schizophrenia. The truth of the matter is that Kraepelin provided page

---

[153]Darrel A. Regier et al., "DSM-5 field trials in the United States and Canada, Part II: Test-retest reliability of selected categorical diagnoses." *American Journal of Psychiatry* 170:59-70 (2013).

after page of clinical description, but no practical or concrete criteria for diagnosing *dementia praecox*.

It was Ewald Hecker's account of hebephrenia, published in 1871, that led Kraepelin to *dementia praecox*. Hecker's comment on the validity of the disease deserves repetition here (it already appears on page 177 of this book). After reporting that a colleague had found no neuropathology in the brain of patient number five, Hecker wrote, "The ultimate evidence that hebephrenia stands as a unitary mental illness in its own right can only be provided by pathologic-anatomic facts. But considering the uncertainty provisionally associated with the pathological anatomy of the brain we probably have to dispense with this proof for a long time." Many people believe that, finally, the time has come to define and diagnose schizophrenia according to its genetic profile and its brain abnormalities. If this could be done, it would strengthen the case for schizophrenia being a natural kind of mental illness.

Alternatively, perhaps it is time to abandon the notion of schizophrenia as a distinct illness. Two distinguished psychiatrists argued just that in a recent article titled, "The slow death of the concept of schizophrenia and the painful birth of the psychosis spectrum."[154] According to them, it would be prudent to return to something like the pre-Kraepelin notion of undifferentiated psychosis, which recognizes a continuous range of symptoms and outcomes. Thus, schizophrenia would be subsumed within a spectrum disorder, in a manner similar to that which has transpired with respect to autism and substance abuse, both of which were previously seen as distinct disorders but which now appear as spectrum disorders in DSM-5.

Assertion No. 4: *Dementia praecox* (schizophrenia) is different from manic-depressive insanity (bipolar disorder)

The identification of *dementia praecox* did not complete Kraepelin's work. It could not have, because once he had identified *dementia praecox* as a distinct illness within the broad, loosely defined group of psychoses, he was obliged to identify other members of that same group. This, of course, is the stuff of classification. Kraepelin, like all intellectually-minded psychiatrists of the nineteenth century, was drawn to classification as a vital component

---

[154]S. Guloksuz and J. van Os, "The slow death of the concept of schizophrenia and the painful birth of the psychosis spectrum." *Psychological Medicine*, 1-16. doi:10.1017/S0033291717001775.

of the sciences they emulated. While zoologists traveled to distant lands looking for, and discovering, new species of animals, psychiatrists visited their asylum wards pondering varieties of mental illness.

The sixth edition of Kraepelin's textbook was the ultimate expression of nineteenth century classification. In this work Kraepelin famously named a new illness, manic-depressive insanity, and in the process he distinguished it from *dementia praecox.* With *dementia praecox* representing disorders associated with a loss of rational thinking, and manic-depressive insanity representing disorders of affect, the whole range of psychoses was effectively partitioned into two large groups. That division was adopted in America and remains evident in DSM-5. Just as *dementia praecox* suffered a number of name changes, so too did manic-depressive insanity. And again, Adolf Meyer had a hand in the changes. As part of his campaign to re-frame mental illnesses as "psychobiological reactions", he introduced the term manic-depressive reaction as a companion to his schizophrenic re-action. Then, in the third edition of the DSM (1980), manic-depressive insanity and manic-depressive reaction were folded into a new diagnostic term, bipolar disorder. While neither of Kraepelin's original disease names is spoken today in the wards of our psychiatric hospitals, his grand parti-tion of psychosis remains in force, now represented by schizophrenia and bipolar disorder.

But, the partition met with opposition in Kraepelin's time, and it is now part of a larger discussion about the usefulness – even the validity – of all psychiatric classifications. Recall that the nineteenth century unitarians denied any categorical distinctions between mental conditions. Kraepelin's contemporary, Alfred Hoche, avoided the word illness altogether, opting instead for symptom complexes, or syndromes. He wrote that the entire exercise of classification was like "trying to clarify a cloudy liquid simply by pouring it from one container into another ... the hopeless pursuit of a mirage."[155]

In America as well, Kraepelin's classification encountered resistance. Adolf Meyer, once a Kraepelin devotee, came to distain it. Karl Men-ninger, the founder of a prominent clinic in Topeka, Kansas, went further. All classifications are nonsense, Menninger said, because the whole notion of mental illness is wrong. In *The Vital Balance* (1919), Menninger wrote, "Gone forever is the notion that the mentally ill person is an exception. It is now accepted that most people have some degree of mental illness at some time, and many of them have a degree of mental illness most of

---

[155]A. Hoche (1912, 1991), pp. 336, 343.

the time."[156] Kraepelin, in his later years, entertained similar thoughts, "Wherever we try to mark out the frontier between mental health and disease, we find a neutral territory, in which the imperceptible change from the realm of normal life to that of obvious derangement takes place."[157]

Current critics of classification understandably target the DSM, which is the custodian of psychiatric diagnosis and classification in North America. In the Spring of 2013, just before the release of the most recent edition, Thomas Insel, then director of the National Institute of Mental Health (United States), posted this surprising statement on his web blog,

> While the DSM has been described as a 'bible' for the field, it is at best, a dictionary, creating a set of labels and defining each. The strength of each of the editions of DSM has been 'reliability' – each edition has ensured that clinicians use the same terms in the same ways. The weakness is its lack of validity. Unlike our definitions of ischemic heart disease, lymphoma, or AIDS, the DSM diagnoses are based on a consensus about clusters of clinical symptoms, not any objective laboratory measure. In the rest of medicine this would be equivalent to creating diagnostic systems based on the nature of chest pain or the quality of fever.[158]

Insel's criticism of the proposed DSM-5 did not stop its publication, but it did encourage other critics. In voicing their concerns about the lack of validity in DSM definitions, commentators pointed out that two individuals with very different symptoms can nonetheless be diagnosed with the same illness. That happens because of the mixed nature of the criteria (their heterogeneity). For example, one person may have delusions and reduced affect, while a second person may have neither of those symptoms but show disorganized speech and reduced motivation. Under DSM-5 guidelines, both persons would be diagnosed with schizophrenia.

It can also happen that a single patient is diagnosed with two or more distinct disorders (comorbidity), owing to an overlap of definitions. An example comes from a major psychiatric center in Houston, Texas where

---

[156] Karl Menninger, *The Vital Balance: The Life Process in Mental Health and Illness.* New York, Viking (1963), p. 33.

[157] Emil Kraepelin, *Lectures on Clinical Psychiatry*, 3rd ed. New York, William Wood (1917), p. 295.

[158] Thomas Insel, https://www.nimh.nih.gov/about/directors/thomas-insel/blog/2013/transforming-diagnosis.shtml (April 29, 2013).

two hundred sixty-four diagnoses were analyzed.[159] Three of the center's most common, single-disorder diagnoses are listed below, together with the percentage of each named diagnosis relative to the total number of diagnoses. Next, the most common multiple diagnoses are listed, with their percentages.

- Posttraumatic stress disorder, 12%

- Major depressive disorder, 10%

- Alcohol use disorder, 8%

- Posttraumatic stress disorder *and* major depressive disorder, 11%

- Posttraumatic stress disorder *and* alcohol use disorder, 9%

- Posttraumatic stress disorder *and* alcohol use disorder *and* major depressive disorder, 7%

These data show that patients were given multiple diagnoses almost as often as single diagnoses, a remarkable result given that each named disorder is supposed to be distinct. It is like saying someone has diabetes *and* cancer – possible, but surely more rare than a patient having one disease *or* the other. The prevalence of multiple diagnoses in psychiatry suggests that some disorders are defined in such a manner that they intersect or overlap with other disorders.

The imprecision of diagnostic criteria generates other types of problems. In one published commentary, the DSM-IV was said to be,

> replete with problematic boundary disputes, many of which could be the result of arbitrary categorical distinctions being imposed along common, underlying domains of functioning. New diagnoses added to the nomenclature ... reflect not so much the discovery of a previously unrecognized disease, pathogen, or lesion but are instead efforts to fill gaps among existing categories.[160]

---

[159]D.A. Regier et al. (2013).

[160]Quotes from Thomas A. Widger and Douglas B. Samuel, "Diagnostic categories or dimensions? A question for the *Diagnostic and Statistical Manual of Mental Disorders – Fifth Edition." Journal of Abnormal Psychology* 114:494-504.

Filling the gaps between "arbitrary categorical distinctions" has led to the inclusion of about three hundred disorders in the latest edition of the diagnostic manual, DSM-5. The difficulty of differentiating related disorders is particularly evident in the area of personality disorders, where the DSM names ten separate disorders. Schizophrenia is another disputed area. Many psychiatrists believe that there are conditions which are "schizophrenia-like", but not actually schizophrenia. As a solution to this problem, the DSM-5 includes "schizoaffective disorder", which is said to be the "prototypic boundary condition" (note 161). First introduced to the DSM in 1980, schizoaffective disorder was meant to cover cases in which a person has symptoms characteristic of *both* schizophrenia (delusions, hallucinations, disorganized thought) *and* mood disorders (depression and mania). The diagnosis of schizoaffective disorder is highly controversial owing to its poor definition, low reliability and overuse.

To investigate whether the diseases schizophrenia, schizoaffective disorder and bipolar disorder are really distinct and if so, in what ways, several prominent psychiatrists formed a research consortium. They began by asking whether each disorder has a unique set of symptoms. Patients were evaluated on a range of symptoms using interviews and clinical tests. The long list of possible symptoms included delusions, hallucinations, disorganized thinking, blunted affect, stereotyped thinking, mania, depression, tension, anxiety and social functioning.

In this manner, a symptom profile was generated for each patient, this being a compilation of his or her test results.

After analysis, it was found that the symptom profiles corresponded only weakly to disease descriptions as defined in the DSM. Patients diagnosed with schizophrenia and patients diagnosed with bipolar disorder shared "a high degree of overlap in clinical characteristics." As for schizoaffective disorder, "Clinical and demographic characteristics ... were often more similar to those of the schizophrenia (patients) than those of the bipolar group ... Yet, in some cases, the characteristics of schizoaffective disorder mirrored those of psychotic bipolar disorder."[161]

So, the consortium asked whether neurobiological measures would work better than psychological and social measures for differentiating between schizophrenia, schizoaffective disorder and bipolar disorder. They considered a variety of measures that had previously been shown to characterize

---

[161]Carol A. Tamminga et al., "Clinical phenotypes of psychosis in the Bipolar-Schizophrenia Network on Intermediate Phenotypes (B-SNIP)." *American Journal of Psychiatry* 170:1263-1274 (2013). Quotes on p. 1269.

one or another of these conditions, among which eye movements, verbal memory, whole brain images, electrical activity in resting brains and physiological responses evoked by auditory stimuli. Unfortunately, these neurobiological measures worked no better than the psychological and social measures. They "did not regularly discriminate individuals with different DSM psychosis diagnoses."[162]

Even Kraepelin, near the end of his life, moderated his earlier opinion that schizophrenia and manic-depressive insanity constitute different diseases. In an article published in 1920, he admitted that the symptoms can be similar.

> We shall have to get accustomed to the notion that our much used clinical checklist does not permit us to differentiate reliably manic-depressive insanity from schizophrenia in all circumstances; and that there is an overlap between the two, which depends on the fact that the clinical signs have arisen from certain antecedent conditions.[163]

Nevertheless, Kraepelin insisted that schizophrenia and manic-depressive insanity have different courses ("irreversible dementia" versus "personalities that remain intact"), and so, "we cannot help but maintain that the two disease processes themselves are distinct." Taken together, these statements suggest that Kraepelin recognized the impracticality of reliable diagnosis, but was not ready to abandon the ultimate goal of identifying "real" disease entities.

If neither symptomatic measures nor neurobiological measure validate Kraepelin's disease categories, what about genetics? Again, studies show considerable overlap. There is no genetic profile that can discriminate between schizophrenia and bipolar disease. Certain specific mutations increase the risk for schizophrenia *and* bipolar disease *and*, in some cases, autism. Family studies also suggest a genetic overlap. If each disease had a different genetic basis, one would expect family histories to have multiple cases of *either* schizophrenia *or* bipolar disease, but not both. That is, If one family member had schizophrenia, other members of the extended family might also have schizophrenia, but none would have bipolar disorder,

---

[162]Carol A. Tamminga et al., "Bipolar and schizophrenia network for intermediate phenotypes: Outcomes across the psychosis continuum." *Schizophrenia Bulletin* 40:S131-S137 (2014), quote on p. S131.

[163]Emil Kraepelin, "The manifestations of insanity," transl. D. Beer. *History of Psychiatry* iii:499-529 (1920, 1992), quote on pp. 528-529.

and the opposite would be true of families touched by bipolar disorder. Research reveals a different picture, however. In studies of family pedigrees, it is often found that families have *both* schizophrenia *and* bipolar disease (in different individuals).

Collectively, the research summarized above points to a number of overlapping features in psychotic mental conditions. This leads us to regard Kraepelin's historic distinction between *dementia praecox* (schizophrenia) and manic-depressive insanity (bipolar disorder) as an unproven hypothesis, one best described as tenuous and contentious in professional circles today. Although both illnesses continue to be diagnosed on a daily basis, serious questions have been raised as to their validity. These concerns need to be addressed because the ultimate purpose of diagnosis is effective treatment. Incorrect diagnoses were not a problem in the nineteenth century because sedatives, baths and bed rests were the only treatments available, and they were administered more or less indiscriminately to patients of all diagnostic descriptions. Today, we have drugs targeted to specific psychiatric disorders, and they are the mainstays of treatment. It is important, therefore, to get the diagnoses right.

Psychiatric medications help some patients but not others, and few patients completely. Individual patients are sometimes prescribed two or more medications, and when this involves a "mood stabilizer" together with an "antipsychotic", it again suggests a blended clinical condition somewhere between schizophrenia and bipolar disorder. Outside of psychiatry, other areas of medicine are moving toward individualized treatments. Cancers, for example, are being defined not by their locations and appearances, but by their genetic and biochemical signatures. Only the latter characterizations allow the selection of medications specifically targeted to the cancers of individual patients. The same type of "precision medicine" is needed in psychiatry.

Most psychiatrists believe that we are now coming to the end of the neo-Kraepelian era, one in which mental illnesses are defined by psychological and behavioral symptoms, conceived as real diseases, and treated according to diagnostic categories. In fact, a new era has already begun, with several options for moving forward.

In one approach, already being pursued by some researchers, the goal is to construct a new kind of classification.[164] It will be based on quantifiable signs and symptoms, such as the size of brain areas, rather than all-or-none

---

[164]Brett A. Clementz et al., "Identification of distinct psychosis biotypes using brain-based biomarkers." *American Journal of Psychiatry* 173:373-384.

judgements, such as the presence or absence of hallucinations. Researchers will look for groups of individuals scoring with extreme measurements on the same set of signs or symptoms. An example might be a group of patients with small hippocampi, structural defects in nerve fibers and inaccurate visual tracking of moving objects. Researchers would assign a label to this particular set of extreme measurements, calling it a "biotype" rather than a mental illness. A different group of patients might have small frontal lobes, reduced brain responses to sensory stimuli and reduced ability to inhibit reactions; this grouping would constitute a second type of biotype. For the project to succeed, it will need to study very many patients and very many healthy persons, and the data will have to analyzed using sophisticated statistical tools. Still, it remains to be seen whether the work will produce a classification more valid or more useful than the DSM.

Meanwhile, a group of researchers at the National Institute of Mental Health (NIMH) in the United States is taking a different approach.[165] If successful, it would eventually eliminate classifications altogether, and even discard the concept of discrete mental illnesses. Like Kraepelin's unitarian critics, these psychiatrists do not believe it is possible – or at least not useful – to name illnesses. Rather than treating mental illnesses, they want to repair specific functional problems.

The first step involves identifying the behavioral and psychological functions necessary for healthy living. Wundt and Kraepelin would have called them processes. So far, the NIMH researchers have targeted responses to fear, responses to reward, habit formation, attention, perception, memory and social communication. The next step will be to study the neural control of these functions using genetic, neurobiological, behavioral and psychosocial tools.

The goal is to discover the mechanisms normally operating in the relevant neural circuits, and how they become damaged. Once this is accomplished, the researchers hope to design therapies for repairing the damage and possibly even preventing it. It is an ambitious project and still in its early stages, but it may one day lead to an entirely different way of diagnosing and treating patients.

Much work remains to be done to refine and implement the ideas outlined above. The very existence of the described projects suggests that psychiatry has a considerable way to go before completing its modernization. It may be firmly established as a medical specialty, and it may be scientific in

---

[165]Bruce N. Cuthbert and Thomas R. Insel, "Toward the future of psychiatric diagnosis: the seven pillars of RDoC." *BMC Medicine* 11:126 (2013).

many respects, but few would argue that it fully meets the needs of its patients. The future of psychiatry is likely to depend on its ability to harness the combined powers of psychology, neuroscience and genetics. It is a lofty ambition, but one already foreseen by Bernhard Gudden, Wilhelm Griesinger, Franz Nissl and Emil Kraepelin.

Suggested Readings

German E. Berrios and Roy Porter, *A History or Clinical Psychiatry.* London, Athlone, 1995.

Santiago Ramón y Cajal, *Recollections of My Life.* Cambridge, MA, MIT, 1989.

Rachel Cooper, *Psychiatry and Philosophy of Science.* Montreal, McGill-Queen's University Press, 2007.

Eric J. Engstrom, *Clinical Psychiatry in Imperial Germany: A History of Psychiatric Practice.* Ithaca, NY, Cornell University Press, 2003.

Peter Gay, *Freud: A Life for Our Time.* New York, W.W. Norton, 1988.

Emil Kraepelin, *Memoirs.* Berlin, Springer-Verlag, 1987.

Richard Noll, *American Madness.* Cambridge, MA, Harvard University Press, 2011.

Scull, Andrew. *Madness in Civilization: A Cultural History of Insanity, from the Bible to Freud, from the Madhouse to Modern Medicine.* Princeton, NJ, Princeton University Press, 2015.

Gordon M. Shepherd, *Foundations of the Neuron Doctrine.* New York, Oxford University Press, 1991.

Edward Shorter, *A History of Psychiatry: From the Era of the Asylum to the Age of Prozac.* New York, John Wiley & Sons, 1997.

Edward Shorter, *A Historical Dictionary of Psychiatry.* New York, Oxford University Press, 2005.

Index